Okay, God...
Really?

God's Love When Life Doesn't Go As Planned

My journey with multiple sclerosis;
my journey with God;
my journey to complete healing

RHONDA HENGST

OKAY, GOD... REALLY? GOD'S LOVE WHEN LIFE DOESN'T GO AS PLANNED

1405 SW 6th Avenue • Ocala, Florida 34471 • Phone 352-622-1825 • Fax 352-622-1875
Website: www.atlantic-pub.com • Email: sales@atlantic-pub.com
SAN Number: 268-1250

Published by Red Mangrove Press: an imprint of Atlantic Publishing Group, Inc.

Library of Congress Cataloging-in-Publication Data

Names: Hengst, Rhonda Sue, author.
Title: Okay, God ... really? : God's love when life doesn't go as planned / by Rhonda Sue Hengst.
Description: Ocala : Atlantic Publishing Group, Inc., 2019. | Summary: "When Rhonda Hengst was diagnosed with Multiple sclerosis, she found strength and love through God"— Provided by publisher.
Identifiers: LCCN 2019031825 (print) | LCCN 2019031826 (ebook) | ISBN 9781620236628 (paperback) | ISBN 9781620236635 (ebook)
Subjects: LCSH: Hengst, Rhonda Sue. | Christian women—Religious life—United States. | Multiple sclerosis—Patients—United States—Biography.
Classification: LCC BR1725.H443 A3 2019 (print) | LCC BR1725.H443 (ebook) | DDC 248.8/61968340092 [B]—dc23
LC record available at https://lccn.loc.gov/2019031825
LC ebook record available at https://lccn.loc.gov/2019031826

Printed in the United States

INTERIOR LAYOUT AND JACKET DESIGN: Nicole Sturk

This book is dedicated with so much love to my family. Especially to my husband, Dan, for choosing to stay with me and keep loving me despite the extremely bumpy road.

To my children, Zac and Shaina, for allowing me the endless pleasure of being your mom. To my parents who raised me with love and put God in my heart, to my sisters who share countless memories and along with their families continue to make more.

And to my grandson, Bennett, your smile, giggles, hugs, and kisses bring so much happiness to me. I may not be the nana I thought I'd be, but may you always know that Nana loves you. My prayer for this book is that it leaves a legacy and you grow up knowing how much God loves you too!

Finally, I dedicate this book to those looking for a miracle who need to be encouraged! Don't give up!

Table of Contents

Preface

When I was a little girl, I had dreams and plans for my future. But I don't remember ever saying, "When I grow up, I want to get married, have kids, have a nice house, be happy, and have multiple sclerosis." Nope, multiple sclerosis was not a part of my plan. Yep, my plans changed! But who can honestly say that their life turned out exactly the way they planned? Who can say that their life is exactly as they wanted it to be?

I know there are many more difficult journeys than mine, and there are also many happier journeys than mine. I also know that whether a journey is filled with hardships or happiness, God's love is always available—free of charge! Read the Bible; God's words are life and health, and they give instructions on how to walk in victory! Believe them, and keep believing, especially when everything around you says that what you believe is just not going to happen. You may feel tempted to, but don't give up. Trust God to guide and protect you when you encounter enemies and evil persistence on your journey. God's word—GOD gives hope! This book begins as a memoir but becomes more of a journal of my discussions with God. And as you read this book, because of how my mind works and because when thoughts would pop into my head and when a memory came to my mind, God would just let me go, and because I'm just a regular person who is not an author and I write as I speak and don't always use proper grammar, I advise you to hang on for dear life. In all seriousness, I ask that we become friends, that you laugh and cry with me, and allow me the honor of sharing my conversations and thoughts with not only God but with YOU!

Chapter 1

Life as I Knew It

Almost everyone knows or has heard of someone with multiple sclerosis. If you don't, you do now. Doctors would define MS as a chronic progressive nervous disorder involving the loss of myelin sheath around certain nerve fibers. I define MS as a disease where the brain is attacked by the immune system. The attack leaves a sclerosis (a scar) on the brain, which causes various symptoms like numbness, fatigue, spasticity, speech problems, and even pain, which then may or may not result in some sort of permanent damage. My three best words that describe multiple sclerosis are 'whenever,' 'wherever,' and 'WHATEVER!'

Soon after I got married, I noticed a pain in my right eye. I thought it was my sinuses; my dad had always had problems with his sinuses. That had to be it…sinuses. A few months of annoying discomfort later, I began to experience some vision loss in that eye.

My journey with multiple sclerosis was beginning, and I had no idea.

I will never forget this one Sunday in December 1987. The same week I lost vision in my right eye, my family went to brunch to celebrate our parents' anniversary. And about that brunch—that was the first time I met Ed, my sister's new boyfriend. Everyone knows not to talk with your mouth full, but I apparently forgot that little tidbit of wisdom and accidentally spit food on him. Great first impression, right? It didn't scare him off, though. Ed still married my sister and has never let me forget that moment in history. Now, Ron, who married my sister Shelly, never reminds me of past embarrassing moments. Ed, I think it's time we get over it!

On the way home from that brunch, I started to feel sick. No, I did not eat too much, and food poisoning never crossed my mind. By the time evening had rolled around, I was throwing up constantly. Dan, my husband, left for work the next morning thinking that I had the flu. By late morning, I was so incredibly weak I could barely move. I knew I needed to go to the doctor. I wasn't able to get a hold of Dan, and I remember so clearly lying on the floor with the phone by my side, calling my sister Robin, who left work and drove me to the doctor.

Between the pain and loss of vision in my eye and now the vomiting, the doctor said that before anything else, he was ordering a CAT scan of my brain to search for tumors.

Whoa, what happened to the sinus problems? 'Hey honey, how was your day? By the way, I might have a brain tumor.' Not exactly the words a husband wants to be greeted with.

I had the CAT scan (computerized axial tomography—basically a detailed x-ray) the next morning. After waiting anxiously all day for the results, we got the call that evening. The test was normal—no tumor.

Wednesday morning, I was still super weak and throwing up. I still thought I had the flu but figured there must be something the doctor could do to stop the vomiting. So again, I called my sister and off we went to the doctor, who gave me a shot for the nausea—FINALLY some relief! He was still concerned about the vision loss, and he made an appointment with an eye doctor for that same afternoon. I think my doctor had an idea of what was going on, but he kept it to himself.

Still being weak, my dad took me to that appointment. The eye doctor immediately diagnosed me with optic neuritis. Back then, they gave a steroid shot directly in the eye for optic neuritis. You heard me—IN THE EYE! First they'd do a shot to numb the eye and then do the steroid injection. In all the 23 years I'd been alive, I had never experienced pain like that. I kept saying the name 'Jesus' over and over again. I held on to the chair so hard that my knuckles went white.

As he injected the steroids into my eye, the doctor asked me if I had experienced any numbing, tingling, or weakness accompanying the vision loss.

No, well maybe weakness, I've been THROWING UP FOR THREE DAYS! Why are you asking me these stupid questions? Just hurry up and get this over with! When will this nightmare end?

I went right to bed when I got home, and that day Dan was greeted by my dad.

After a couple weeks of rest, I recovered with only a little bit of vision loss. Dan was only just beginning to experience the 'in sickness and in health' vows we had made to each other such a short time before.

When I was younger, I wanted to have four kids—a boy, another boy, a girl, and then a boy, in that order. That is what I thought I wanted. We were blessed and had Zachary Daniel in 1989. Nineteen months later, we were blessed again with Shaina Marie. I figured that a good time to have another baby was when both kids were in school, but when that came around, the discussion of having more kids didn't really come up. Dan and I found ourselves quite happy with our two, we each could handle one— they couldn't take us. The thought of having four kids had totally fizzled from my mind. And after all, we had the million-dollar family. At least that's what people would tell us. Dan insists that's a joke, he's never gotten his million; he's still waiting.

Seriously though, I remember the thrill of excitement when the doctor said, "It's a girl," when Shaina was born. We never found out the sex and I was positive that this baby was a boy. We did agree on a boy name, but could not agree on a girl name. Then, when Dan gently held this precious black and blue baby (the umbilical cord had been around her head) close to his face and I heard the magical words: "Hello, Shaina Marie. This is your daddy," another thrill of excitement coursed through my veins—it was the girl name I had wanted. Dan says we named her Shaina because I always get my way. WHATEVER!

The last family vacation we took before our lives changed was a trip to Sea World in Ohio. Sometimes, I would wish that I just could go back to that little getaway and to the life we had then. I remember everything about that trip—how much Shaina loved jumping in and out of the water for what seemed like hours at the hotel pool, Zac getting all excited when we'd get splashed at a show, the kids feeding the ducks. But what I remember most is how happy and carefree we were. Dan and I loved each other and our time with our children. Life was good. I was healthy.

Later that same year, I was talking with a co-worker about her sister who had been sick. In passing, she said something that would change my life forever.

"My sister is being tested for multiple sclerosis because she has optic neuritis."

I sat there listening to her talk but didn't hear her. Her voice faded like a radio being turned down. All I could hear were my thoughts screaming at me.

What did she just say? What does she mean it's a symptom of multiple sclerosis? That can't be right. I had optic neuritis! MS. MS. MS. MS. MS.

I couldn't get it out of my head. I can't remember if I said anything to her at the time, but I do remember my heart plunging through the floor. I went home from work that day and called the eye doctor right away.

They told me that optic neuritis could be a symptom of MS, but it wasn't the case all of the time.

Why, why, WHY had they not told me this when they diagnosed me? Seriously, WHY?!

I was feeling more and more anxious by the second. It was as if someone had pushed the panic button inside my head. They seemed to notice the frustration and pure terror in my voice because they quickly told me that the doctor doesn't say anything if the patient has no other symptoms.

Okay, I guess that's a good reason, but still!

I remembered the doctor asking me questions about numbing and tingling. It all made sense. It had been years since my optic neuritis diagnosis.

Rhonda, relax.

I shared with them how I still had no symptoms of MS.

Take a deep breath.

They said that I shouldn't worry and told me that I was probably in the clear.

You're fine.

After hanging up, I sat down in the chair in the kitchen, and my head started spinning.

Wait… PROBABLY? What did they mean 'probably?' That's not good enough!

The panic was back. I didn't want a "probably," I wanted a definite "all clear!" I wanted to hear: "No, you will never have multiple sclerosis."

I had a husband and two young children to think about. Multiple sclerosis couldn't happen—it was *not* in my plans.

It is amazing how the mind works. Each day it became easier and easier to convince myself that I had MS. I was walking to my neighbor's house one day and I thought my legs felt numb. I hadn't been diagnosed. I had no other symptoms. I had never had any tingling or numbness. Yet, here I was, lying on my neighbor's couch, letting my imagination go out of control and convince myself that my legs were numb.

Before I go any farther dear reader, on the off chance you had or currently have optic neuritis and this is the first time you've heard it mentioned that it can sometimes be accompanied by multiple sclerosis, I want to give you a little advice that I wish someone had given me: FORGET ABOUT IT! GET IT OUT OF YOUR HEAD! REBUKE THE THOUGHT IN JE-SUS' NAME!

The kids probably don't remember how I was during that time of uncertainty, but I'm sure Dan does. I was crying a lot. I was scared and depressed. And whether my jag lasted a few weeks or months, it was too long and not good. Dan had his own emotions to deal with, and a crying wife only made everything worse. I look back on that time now and see how the devil works on our minds. Give the devil an inch, and evil takes a mile.

I grew up in a Christian home with two sisters and parents whom I adore and who will always love me. I was fortunate to grow up with God. I know my relationship with Him helped me during that difficult time. God helped me regain my life, and I was happy again. Though I overcame the depression and fear and did stop crying, multiple sclerosis was never far from my mind.

One morning a few years later, I woke up with another problem in the same eye that had optic neuritis. I had no pain like before—only blurriness when I moved my eye. I remember we went to see the movie *Titanic* with friends, and my eyes had to be closed when I turned my head or I would get extremely dizzy. This time, my doctor didn't send me to an eye doctor but to a neurologist. The neurologist thought it would be a good idea to do an MRI. If I had multiple sclerosis, different treatments were now available. There was no cure and the treatment would only help slow the progression of the disease, but there were options now.

When the MRI showed spots on my brain, they diagnosed me with multiple sclerosis.

For me, it's usually easy to recall the timing of events in my life by thinking back to the ages of my kids. I remember the night I was diagnosed very clearly. Zac was in second grade and Shaina was in first grade. There was a Fun Night at their school. All things considered, it was actually a really fun night.

Don't you just love school Fun Nights? We sure did! The cakewalk was the best part; Zac and Shaina would do it until they won. We always had at least one cake to take home. One year, Zac dressed head-to-toe like a cowboy in a hat, boots, and vest—he was adorable. I think that was the same year my dad played the raffle and won the stereo he gave to us. I liked the raffle almost as much as the cakewalk. With this raffle, you always won something, so there was never any disappointment. Dan usually had a headache by the end of the night, most likely due to all the money we went through playing the raffle. Oh well, it was for a good cause.

Anyway, I can remember eating a barbecue in the gym at Fun Night, discussing the diagnoses with my mom. I told her that there was no need to worry and it was going to be okay! I had already processed the shock and fear when I had freaked out over the possibility of a diagnosis years ago. Now that it was a reality, it was nothing new, and I really was okay with it. I believed multiple sclerosis was God's plan for my life.

Thankfully, they no longer gave steroid shots in the eye. My eye was still having nightmares! They now delivered the medicine intravenously. I began the first of many outpatient steroid treatments at the hospital and then started a multiple sclerosis treatment the following summer. My loving husband gave me my weekly injection. Dan hated needles. He always passed out when getting his blood drawn, but here he was giving his wife a shot. With a long needle. I always made sure to be nice to Dan on shot day.

There are different types of multiple sclerosis, and MS has many symptoms. There are similarities, but most people are affected differently. I happened to be symptom-free for years, for which I am very thankful. This was also very convenient for me since I loved volunteering at the kids' school. I remember when the symptoms first started. I was healthy and walking normally when I went with Zac on his fourth grade end-of-the-year field trip. It was the next year that I started having problems with my balance and began to experience weakness in my legs. The symptoms came so quietly, like a wolf in sheep's clothing. I got a walker to use at home but preferred to just hold on to someone else when we were in public. Oh yes, another job for Dan.

Dan would say that I had gotten multiple sclerosis just to get him to hold my hand. Yep, Dan was right. This had all been to get him to hold my hand. Good for him—he figured something out about me.

I also had braces made for both my legs, which helped tremendously with the drop foot that had developed. It was during Zac's sixth-grade year that we bought a wheelchair. At first I absolutely hated it. I would only use the wheelchair if I knew I was in for a lot of standing or walking. But as the weakness became a daily reminder of the multiple sclerosis in my life, the wheelchair became my gift from God, it not only gave me freedom, but also my husband, and I loved it! I appreciated the freedom it gave Dan, he said he felt like a weirdo just hanging out by the ladies restroom, and since it would appear that most women have conversations in the restroom, and me being as I am, poor guy, Dan was always waiting for me.

By the time both kids were in middle school, volunteering opportunities had started to diminish, but I was able to work the candy store every year. I went with a purse full of change and a good book to fill the time. Zac and Shaina ate their lunch as quickly as they could so they could spend the rest of the period visiting me. Whether they came to see their mom or because I bought them something each and every time, it didn't matter to me—I just loved spending time with them. But either way they never seemed embarrassed of their wheelchair-bound mother. In fact, they actually seemed proud of me. When they'd walk past the store between classes, Zac and Shaina would yell, "I love you, Mom," or swing in for a quick hug, never caring who heard or saw. Middle-school-aged kids showing their mother public affection. The principal even made a comment about that. I am not exaggerating. Okay, I am bragging, but not exaggerating. All I'm gonna say about that is…let me have a moment to reminisce in my mind about those wonderful, happy times.

Working the candy store was one of my favorite memories of when the kids were in middle school. I really enjoyed it. I would drive to school and Zac would get out of class and meet me in the parking lot where he'd get the wheelchair out of the trunk and help me set up the candy store. After the final lunch period, he'd get out of class again to help close the candy store and put my wheelchair back in the car. I think that's when Zac really started to find perks with the MS—getting out of class was a big perk. I can say this now—it was pretty obvious that Zac took his sweet time helping me.

Shaina also helped with the candy store, but I don't think she saw it as much as a perk—at least not at first. But that could have something to do with a slightly bad experience she had. Shaina was a rather shy sixth grader and was more than a little nervous about her first time helping me with the store. Zac had told her not to worry—she'd be excused, it was easy, she could do it. As I sat in the car waiting for Shaina to come help me, I looked at my watch, noticing that it was getting later and later. I thought that maybe she had forgotten, so I decided to get out of the car on my own. It took a little longer than it would have with help. Getting the wheelchair out of the trunk was difficult and I could have hurt myself, but I managed.

I had made it into the candy store when Shaina ran in with tears streaming down her face. She apologized and explained that when she asked her teacher if she could come help me, he had said no.

Really? He wouldn't let her leave class a few minutes early to help her disabled mom who was volunteering to help the school? Okay, he must have his reasons, but really?

Shaina said that she was so worried for me. My heart broke for this precious child who was standing in front of me so visibly upset. I hugged her tightly and assured her that it was no problem—I was fine.

Later on, when Dan came home from work, I started crying. The more I thought about how upset my daughter had been, the more I cried. As I was explaining to him what happened, Shaina came home from school and *she* was crying. Dan took one look at his sobbing wife and daughter, and left. As the door closed behind him, Shaina and I looked at each other and smiled for the first time that afternoon. We knew where he was going. You see, Dan has this look that can be intimidating, and some may even say scary. Who am I kidding—he IS intimidating. He may not think so, oh, but he is and can be. Needless to say, Shaina never had to worry again about getting out of class. When we talk about this story, we no longer cry, we laugh at the thought of Dan confronting the teacher.

The memories of those middle school years will forever be embedded in my head and engraved on my heart. I still don't think my kids are embarrassed or ashamed of me. Now they just get annoyed with me. So PLEASE let me have my moment.

Both Zac and Shaina were active all throughout high school. And the wheelchair totally became my gift from God. Dan and I even found a multiple sclerosis perk when Zac was on the golf team: we always got to follow Zac in a golf cart as he golfed. Everyone else had to walk the nine or 18 holes if they wanted to watch a player. I know those who could walk were lucky and it was good exercise, but at that moment I loved riding in the cart and feeling the breeze when it was hot or having a blanket wrapped around me when it was cold. Funny story: once, as my mom and I watched Zac play, we thought the cart was having a problem because it wouldn't stop vibrating. We tried everything to get it to stop, but no matter what, it vibrated. What was wrong with this cart? Then I realized that my cell phone was vibrating in my purse. It wasn't the cart, it was my phone! Silence is expected on the golf course, but we could not stop laughing.

I really did feel like my wheelchair was a gift from God. One time, Dan and I were in a store when an older gentlemen explained that his wife needed a wheelchair and was waiting for one of the store's chairs to become available. I must look like a therapist because he kept talking and went on to explain that he and his wife never went anywhere or did anything because she was too embarrassed to use a wheelchair. Boy, I needed to talk to this woman! I found his wife at the front of the store. I wheeled up to her and introduced myself. I explained that using a wheelchair is nothing to be embarrassed about and that she shouldn't let it get in the way of enjoying life with her husband. I told her that wheelchairs are gifts from God—mine certainly was. We chatted a little while longer before she and her husband left, both smiling.

As much as a gift my wheelchair was, I wasn't able to use it in the house because of the stairs and doorways. When my legs felt too weak for the walker, I would just fall to my knees and crawl or scoot across the floor. It was excellent for the biceps and my abs but terrible for the knees and my jeans. That does explain the patches on all of my jeans. Dan even bought me a pair of kneepads for Christmas one year. This was how it went at our house. When I was tired and I didn't have much strength, I would crawl. When I was extremely tired, Dan would pick me up and carry me like a child. I could wrap my arms around his neck and whisper sweet nothings in his ear—it didn't happen, but it could have. Dan was my favorite gift from God. Later on, when he had gotten older, I also had Zac. Being his mom and not wanting the sweet nothings, Zac's way did the job, but it made me a little nervous. Zac would just grab ahold of me around my knees and throw me over his shoulders like I was a bag of potatoes.

When I began using the wheelchair most of the time except for when I crawled around the house, I decided to stop wearing the braces. They hurt my legs and made it nearly impossible to crawl. Now that I wasn't walking as much, there really wasn't a need for them. It never even occurred to me that the multiple sclerosis was progressing and I wasn't sad about it. In fact, I even felt a little bit excited. I would be able to wear normal shoes again. It had been hard to find shoes that fit the braces. I was so excited to finally wear cute shoes again—SANDALS! I could wear sandals again. As I think about that now I find it interesting—I'm not even a shoe person.

Dan had been feeling uneasy about me driving with a drop foot. I don't know why. I thought I was driving fine. He might have felt uneasy because I used my hand to lift my leg from the gas to the brakes and back again. But really, it worked fine. To humor my husband, I stopped driving when Zac started—Dan won that one. It wasn't all bad; I got to have my own personal driver. That's when Zac discovered another perk of having a mother with multiple sclerosis. Besides using the MS to get his driving permit earlier than the rest of the class—yes he did—he also found handicapped parking to be a great perk.

After being diagnosed, I would say to my friends, "I can handle this. I just don't want any symptoms." And I was symptom-free for many years. But that eventually changed. Then I remember saying, "I can handle this. I just don't want my symptoms to get any worse." But that also eventually changed. I know it was by the Grace of God that I was able to still handle it.

Over the years, my relationship with God strengthened and I fell deeper and deeper in love with Him. I learned how to recognize His voice. God can speak in many ways, but He often speaks to me through my thoughts. God will speak to my spirit and then my spirit will speak to my mind. Then suddenly, I have a new thought.

I will always remember the first noticeable thought I received from God. It was spring and we had just gotten home from a baseball game during Zac's last year of Little League. I went in the living room with a glass of pop and some pretzels, all set to relax after a fun morning. As soon as I sat down, it occurred to me that I had walked up the three stairs to get into the kitchen normally.

Did I just walk up the steps normally?

Steps were difficult for me.

I didn't use the handrail, did I?

I sat stunned. Suddenly, the thought occurred to me to get up and walk. I knew it was more than a thought. I told Zac that I needed to walk. He didn't question me (those sure were the days). We went outside, and I started walking unassisted up and down the back part of the driveway.

I hadn't walked by myself for quite a while, so Zac walked backwards in front of me in case he needed to catch me.

Dan was gone at the time and came home to find me standing in the driveway, holding onto the basketball hoop. When he asked what I was doing, I told him to watch. I walked to him and paced in circles around him, completely unassisted. I had no balance problems and I felt completely strong. Dan smiled, swept me up into a hug, and swung me around. We kissed and cried tears of joy, totally forgetting the kids were there. Okay, we didn't forget the kids were there and there was no swinging, but it was a beautiful moment. I totally believed with all my heart that I had been healed—we all did.

By evening, I was back to being unable to walk on my own. But I wasn't discouraged. We all knew what happened. It wasn't a dream—it was real. I wasn't in remission; there was no new MS drug, no new steroid treatment, no new anything. The only possible explanation was God! It had all come from a thought. If I hadn't listened to and obeyed that thought, I would have missed an incredible miracle.

Over the course of the next few weeks, I had several more thoughts to get up and walk. I obeyed, and I walked. But then one day it stopped and almost a year passed before it happened again. Out of the blue one night while I was sitting by the computer, another thought occurred to me to walk. Dan was sleeping on the couch in the living room and Shaina was in bed. Zac was the only one awake, so I called him. He sat on the counter in the kitchen and cheered me on while I walked back and forth from the sink to the fridge without hanging onto anything. My walking miracles never lasted very long. I would say that they were my glimpses from God that I would one day be healed. God was giving me a taste of what he could do. Dan liked to say that it was time for me to get the whole meal—I couldn't help but agree.

I've experienced many miracles and what I call 'God moments' since being diagnosed with multiple sclerosis. A lot of them seemed to involve my head. I do remember a head miracle happening before my MS symptoms began. One day, with no explanation, before any symptoms of MS, I fell right in front of Zac and Shaina in the kitchen and hit my head hard on the stove. I got up and touched my head. I wasn't exactly sure what just happened, but my head didn't hurt. The kids were so worried that I had hurt myself, but no bruise ever developed. Another miracle happened when I tripped over a rug in my bedroom and barely missed hitting my head on the wall. That time I was lucky. Another time, though, I wasn't as lucky and tripped on the same rug and fell flat on my chin (you're probably thinking that I should have moved the rug, but I liked it there). Dan and Zac were in the room at the time and rushed to my side. I lifted my chin off the floor, and I could see in Dan's eyes that we were going to the hospital to get stitches. Plus, Dan told me that we were going to the hospital. I never hurt myself when I hit the back of my head, the time I fall forward... stitches. God must want to protect my brain cells.

Come to think of it, God has been protecting my brain cells for a long time. I was hit by a car when I was 14. I had gone to my High School State Honors Choir tryouts. My friends and I had made the choir and were having a good day UNTIL the driver of the van made the mistake of dropping me off on the street in front of my house instead of pulling in the driveway and I made the mistake of crossing the street behind the van instead of in front of it. I remember waiting for one car, then BAM. I never saw the car coming. The bumper hit my legs, and my shoulder smashed the windshield as I flew over the top of the car and landed on the side of the road.

The couple that hit me felt terrible, but it wasn't their fault. I was in the emergency room waiting to go into surgery for my shoulder when my sister wheeled the wife of the man who had hit me into my room in a wheelchair. She wasn't hurt—just extremely shaken up. She needed to see with her own eyes that I was not only alive and breathing, but also okay mentally. Both she and her husband believed that it had been my head that had hit the window. Nope, it wasn't my head—God was protecting my brain cells. After I recovered, the nice couple had me over for dinner a few of times. I think I needed to help them recover.

I had several God moments with that accident, my favorite was being carried by angels over the top of the car and being set down gently on the side of the road where they found me. I was just sitting there, and I wasn't in any pain. I couldn't see anything. They found my glasses on the other side of the road (unbroken and with no scratches—phew!). Even though I had landed in gravel, I had no scratch either and my clothes were fine. All except my blouse, that is. It was my mom's favorite blouse she had let me borrow. I can still see my mom in the emergency room at the hospital convincing me that it was all right for them to cut the blouse off because my shoulder was so swollen. I will never forget that, and I will for sure always love the story about the angels carrying me, and so will my mom.

Another God moment happened one morning while I was attempting to shower. Our bathroom had a combination tub and shower, which meant that I had to lift my leg up over the edge of the tub to get into the shower. I tried three times but was unsuccessful each time. I simply could not find the strength or the balance to lift my leg up and get in. As I rested on the toilet seat before making yet another attempt, I shouted, "God, come on! I just want to TAKE A SHOWER!"

I shouldn't have yelled, but I was frustrated. All I wanted to do was take a simple shower. God understood and heard me because when I tried again, I made it into the shower easily—more proof, as if more was needed, that God was listening and with me at all times.

In February of Zac's tenth grade year and Shaina's ninth grade year, I was hospitalized unexpectedly for six days. I had been scheduled to have outpatient surgery on a Tuesday (nothing serious, no need to get personal, it was just a choice to have a female procedure). The Sunday before the scheduled procedure, I began having horrible pains in my stomach. I spent a long day and night in the emergency room as they tested for everything under the sun to explain my stomach distress. They thought it was possibly appendicitis, but they weren't sure. We had arrived at the ER around 1 in the afternoon, but when 2 am rolled around and they still were not positive what was happening, Dan walked to the nurses station and politely informed them that we were leaving. Enough was enough—I was

EXHAUSTED and needed to get home, take my MS injection, and go to bed. He explained that we lived close by and could return right away when they had a diagnosis. Remember how I mentioned that Dan could have an intimidating look? Well, let's just say that they didn't dare to argue with him at that point. We left the hospital.

When we arrived back home, Dan crawled into bed. While I was in the bathroom taking out my contacts, I had a little discussion with God. It wasn't to thank him that I was okay; it was more an explanation to him that I didn't want anyone to think I made this up. Dan never complained, but I did explain to God how bad I felt that Dan had wasted a Sunday afternoon. After our discussion, I went to the bedroom and I, too, crawled into bed. And, no joke, as soon as my head hit the pillow, Dan barely asleep, the phone rang. They had finally had a diagnosis. Less than 20 minutes after we'd left to go home, we were back at the hospital with me in my pajamas! Thanks, God! It wasn't all in my head. Does this mean I have to thank God for the surgery that is needed?

Early Monday morning, I had my appendix out. They kept me overnight, and I had my scheduled procedure on Tuesday morning as planned. As ecstatic as I was to have everything done with—Dan might be right about me getting my way—when I woke up in the recovery room, it didn't take long for me to decide that I probably should have rescheduled the other procedure. Being under two days in a row had an effect on me and I could hardly move one part of my body. Neither surgeon knew what to do, so they called the neurologist. Within minutes, the neurologist said that I'd be staying in the hospital for at least four more days. I was going to start IV steroids twice a day along with physical therapy.

A wave of depression and panic washed over me as they wheeled me into my hospital room.

WHAT? Are you kidding me? I can't be here four more days! My family will think that it's nicer not having me at home. They will realize their life is much easier without me. Oh no, the thoughts are starting. Zac and Shaina aren't

*going to miss me at all! They'll say 'Mom who?' Dan will think that he wants a
healthy wife. This is horrible!*

Once again the devil and my thoughts were running wild. Shaina could tell
something was wrong so she wrote 'I love you, Mom' on the marker board
in my hospital room. I knew my family loved me, but that didn't change
how I was feeling. I was crabby and sad—I was pitiful! After insisting that
Dan and the kids leave, which they did, the devil continued having fun in
my mind. I cried myself to sleep, feeling completely defeated.

For Christmas that year, my mom had gotten me Joel Olsteen's book,
"Your Best Life Now." I had Dan include it with a few things he brought
from home. I thought the time I spent in the hospital might be good time
to start reading it. God must have thought so too because I woke up at 4
am, opened the book, and began to read.

It didn't take long for me to totally understand why I was in that hospital
room. I needed to rest and take time to focus on the one who has promised in Isaiah 40:31 that "those who wait on the Lord shall renew their
strength." My whole attitude changed immediately as I read. The urge to
call Dan came over me. I HAD to talk to him. My family had left so badly
the night before, but it was still way too early. I waited as long as I could
and called the house at 6:30 am. I woke him up, but he didn't seem to
mind. He might have been a little frightened but not bothered. I told him
that I loved him and that I didn't want him to worry about me—I was going to be just fine. I asked him to please tell the kids the same. I was kind
and loving. I was nice. I'm quite sure that Dan did not fall back to sleep after that unexpected phone call but he probably passed out from the shock.

After I hung up, I kept reading and read that if I looked hard enough and
kept the right attitude, I could find something good in any experience. I
knew that doing that would be hard in a lot of situations, but I could do
my best in this one, at least. For the following four days, I was at a spa in
my mind. I pushed a button and someone would come see what I wanted.
I received as many back rubs as I wanted. I had the bed, pillows, blankets,
and television all to myself. I could turn the light and TV on whenever I

wanted, even at night. Question: why is it that a man can fall asleep with the lights and TV on, but when he goes to bed, they have to be off immediately so he can sleep? Just curious! Anyway, I had 24-hour room service, with three meals a day, dessert included. And, believe it or not, this hospital actually had good food. Dan and the kids ate there every day. Dan was also finding good in this situation—he didn't have to plan meals.

Side story: When Dan asked my parents for my hand in marriage, they warned him that I didn't know how to cook. Dan assured them that we would learn together. Dan learned—I'm still learning, and my parents are still laughing. Dan became the preferred chef in the family. Both of Dan's parents are cooks, so it is no surprise that Dan enjoys cooking and is good at it. Dan says he cooks out of necessity; if he wants to eat, he has to cook. Whatever!

While it got easier to control my attitude, I had no control over how chatty the steroids made me. People laughed at me. Not with me, AT me! Zac teasingly made comments about how his mom was on 'roids. I couldn't really get bothered by that statement because I *was* having massive doses of steroids pumped in my body twice a day intravenously. Those four days went by quickly. What could have been a depressing stay in the hospital turned into an amazing experience with God that I will never forget. God renewed my strength as He promised, and by the end of the week, I was up and walking with a walker.

I went home on Saturday, but because the doctor said I shouldn't try and climb stairs after the appendectomy, and since our bedroom was upstairs, I had to spend the next week upstairs. My first night back at home, Shaina and I were chatting in my bedroom. She asked if I was glad to be home because she said I seemed depressed. I told her that I was very glad to be home. And there was no place else I'd rather be. But I had to admit that I was feeling a little down. I had just spent the last four days with God, talking to Him whenever I wanted and talking about Him to whoever would listen. I had never before felt so totally filled with God. After Shaina left the bedroom, it became clear to me that I wanted and needed this time upstairs. I needed an opportunity to come down from the high I was on. I needed time to process all that God had put into my heart. And to be honest, I craved more alone time with God. I didn't go downstairs even once that entire week. By the end of the week, I felt much stronger and was ready to once again love God and be a wife and mother at the same time.

One morning as Dan was getting ready for work, I told him that God must have something for me to do after the experience I had. That same morning, I was sitting on the toilet and looking out the window of the bathroom when all of a sudden, it was supernaturally that I knew what God meant for me to do. I needed to speak to women and encourage them by sharing what all I had been learning from this experience. I called my mom and a few of my friends and talked to them about what God wanted me to do. I wasn't scared! I was excited! God knew I liked to talk—that was certainly not the problem. Obviously because of the excitement I wasn't thinking clearly—talking in front of people who would be looking at me would be a problem. I was nervous just thinking about it and fear showed up.

No, public speaking and nerves do not go together. When I'm nervous, my mind goes blank, I lose my train of thought, and my mind will wander and go in several directions at once. I struggle getting to the point and have random thoughts, and that's not all. I also talk way faster than normal. What's more, I tend to get emotional when talking about God, and public speaking while crying doesn't seem like a good time. Oh my, yes, fear showed up!

Dan said that as long as I spoke from the heart, I'd be fine. But I didn't want to take any chances. Knowing how my mind works, I decided to write down what I wanted to say beforehand and read from the heart. I sat down at the computer and typed word for word what I wanted to say. I even wrote, "Hi, I'm Rhonda," in one of the versions.

We went to a sports award night for our kids soon after the incredible God week. There's a hall in the school that is all windows, so at night, it looked like a hall of mirrors. I saw my husband pushing me in the wheelchair in the reflection of the windows and I felt different. I had a defining moment. People are watching me. I might be in a wheelchair, but I need to look my best, hold my head up, and keep a smile on my face because I represent God!

But the thought of standing up and talking in front of people still made me nervous. I thought of asking everyone to close their eyes and just listen while I talked. Or I could be in the next room with a microphone—that would work too. And it has to be said—the MS probably doesn't help, but my mind worked this way years prior to any MS symptom. I talked so fast in an 8th grade musical's speaking part that no one knew what I had said, and 'Tizzy' was a nickname in high school.

Really, God? You want me to speak in public? Okay, God... Really?

Despite the nerves that seemed to be snowballing, I discovered that I loved to write. I felt like it brought me incredibly close to God. As much as I loved writing though, it wasn't long before my husband began expressing his irritation with how often I was on the computer rewriting the speech. I went through so much ink and paper. I bounced ideas off of the same women's group from my church at least three separate times. They were a fabulous group of women who let me treat them like guinea pigs. My dear friend Pam was led to drive and I spoke—we would joke that we felt like Moses and Aaron, a team working for God. But as much as I enjoyed the writing part, I kept finding excuses to put off the actual speaking part.

A year and a half went by when another plan changed. Dan had taken me out for dinner for our 20th wedding anniversary, and as soon as we sat down, he looked deep into my eyes and said, "You're not the only one God has been speaking to. He has been speaking to me too. God told me that you need to write a book." Had I just heard him correctly? I thought he was going to express his undying love for me, but that's not what I heard. Dan was usually a very private person when it came to his faith, so after I asked him to repeat what he said a few times, I knew I heard correctly—this was real.

Of course! I can write a book! I would much rather write a book about my journey than speak in public—no fear would be involved. Finally—a plan that changed for the better!

Now Dan encourages me to be on the computer. Oh, and later that night Dan did express his undying love for me.

Chapter 2

My Speech—A Stepping Stone

When I sat down to write this book, I started out by reading through all the speeches I had saved on my computer. In my fourth version of the speech, I wrote: "God could have asked me to write a book—that would have been a little easier on the nerves."

Wow, MORE proof that God is real. By telling Dan, He was including both of us in this new plan. I see my speech as a stepping stone, a step that was obviously needed on my journey.

My speech was such an important part of my journey with multiple sclerosis and with God that I feel like I need to share it with you. So here it is, just as the speech was written. I've got to tell you how good it feels that you're the one reading it and not me!

My Unedited Speech

My husband came home from a meeting in Chicago and suggested I start my little talks (little talks?) with this question: On a scale of 1 to 10, what value were you when you were born? What value do you feel you are today? You are still 10s. You have the same value to God now as you did when you were born.

Nobody, especially not God, ever said life would be easy. Jesus didn't say "if" we have trouble, He said we WILL have trouble. There is pain, suffering, and many struggles in life. Because of sin. The devil brought the sin in the world.

The devil IS the sin in the world. The devil's very much alive and all around us. God makes it very clear that the devil's intentions are to kill, steal, and destroy. Our struggles aren't with God—our struggles are with the devil. The Bible tells us to be self-controlled and alert because the devil is as a roaring lion looking for someone to devour. We do need to be alert because as long as we have breath, the devil will do whatever he can to attack us. We have to do whatever we can to resist him. In the Bible, Paul gives great advice: he tells us to put on the full armor of God so that we can take our stand against the devil's schemes. God's armor will help in the fight to resist the devil. My suggestion—read Ephesians 6 and PUT IT ON!

When I was first diagnosed with multiple sclerosis, the doctor compared multiple sclerosis to playing a game of darts. The doctor said the brain is the dartboard, the attacks are the darts. With multiple sclerosis the brain is attacked with lesions, like someone throwing darts at a dartboard. I remember the doctor saying, "You never know when or if a dart will hit the bullseye." The King James Bible says the shield of faith will protect you from the fiery darts from the evil one. Needless to say the shield of faith became my much-needed favorite piece of armor. You know, we have a dartboard in our family room. I've never hit the bullseye. Purely physiological. Oh, I could if I wanted to. I just don't want to.

The shield of faith may be my favorite, but I fall more in love with the sword of the spirit every day. We have incredible power with the sword. The sword of the spirit is the word of God; the word of God is the Bible. The Bible says in John 1:14 that "the word became flesh and made his dwelling among us." The Bible is Jesus. His name alone has more power and authority than most people realize. When the devil attacks (because he will), say the name 'Jesus' and visualize yourself throwing the Bible at him. Not in a disrespectful way to God's word, but in a hurtful way to the devil. It's great to throw God's promises at Satan. He must hate that. Sometimes I'll say the name 'Jesus' over and over and over again. Visualizing the devil crouched in a corner with his hands over his head totally works for me. YEP, the devil hates the power we have in God's word. He knows Jesus came to destroy his works. And you know what? You can put your armor on and resist the devil with confidence, because Jesus DID destroy his works. Jesus defeated the devil on the cross.

I want to learn all I can about God. We need to have a teachable spirit. I feel like the best way for me to learn is to be in God's word, myself, every day. I know the Bible can be hard to understand. There is so much in the Bible that people of God interpret differently. It is hard to know who or what to believe. My advice is to not get caught up in the arguing that happens with Christians about what they believe. The Bible says in Titus 3:9, "But avoid foolish controversies and genealogies and quarrels about the law, because these are unprofitable and useless." The Message version says that quarreling is unprofitable and will get you nowhere. It's pretty clear God doesn't want us to argue. Again, my suggestion is to search the scriptures for yourself and let the word of God speak to you personally. Let God speak to you and believe what God puts in your heart to believe.

Many people think that everything, good and bad, only comes from God. As totally understandable as that may be, I personally don't believe God gave me multiple sclerosis, which I do call bad…really bad. Now, this would be a topic Christians argue about. I don't want to argue and I'm not trying to offend anyone, I just really feel this needs to be said, this topic IS something God spoke to me about, so please let me explain why I believe the way I do. My earthly father loves me so much. He doesn't want me to have this disease. My dad wouldn't give me this disease to punish me or to teach me something. He would NEVER give me this disease to get me to spend more time with him. How could I believe that God, my heavenly father, who loves me SO MUCH MORE than my earthly father, would EVER deliberately give me something that would hurt me? Saying and believing God gave me multiple sclerosis makes my dad sound cruel and mean. I don't want to see my dad that way and I am NOT going to see my God that way.

There's a story in the Bible about a crippled woman Jesus healed. The Pharisees were upset Jesus healed this woman on the Sabbath. Jesus didn't care. Jesus said in Luke 13:16, "Then should not this woman—a daughter of Abraham, whom Satan has kept bound for eighteen long years, be set free on the Sabbath day from what bound her?" Jesus didn't say God gave her the infirmity, he said she was bound by Satan. In Acts 10, Peter is discussing Jesus at a house in Caesarea. In verse 38, Peter says, "How God anointed Jesus of Nazareth with the Holy Spirit and power, and how he went around doing good and healing all who were under the power of the devil, because God was with him." The Bible says Jesus went around and healed all those who were under the power of the DEVIL.

I was excited to share my speech with a couple of special people in my life. When said I believed God didn't give me multiple sclerosis, they became mad at me. They felt I was taking God's control and giving power to the devil. I understood what they were saying, but it hurt they didn't let me explain what I was saying. I'm not nor would I ever take God's control. No one is more powerful than God—NO ONE. For me, it's not about God's control, it's about God's LOVE. A comment was made about not wanting to give the devil credit. I have a hard time with the word "credit" and "devil" in the same sentence—credit is positive, right? We want to have good credit. Multiple sclerosis isn't positive or good. God doesn't want credit for multiple sclerosis, the devil can have the blame for that. Lying in bed that night, I remember feeling so sad. I never did get to share my speech with them. I haven't to this day. I'm not saying the devil attacked and gave me multiple sclerosis. Maybe he did, maybe he didn't. I don't know. But I do know we are born and live in a fallen world, and God didn't create a fallen world. God didn't create a world with sin or sickness. God created a PERFECT world. God even said it was very good. Who am I hurting by believing God didn't give me multiple sclerosis? Seriously, who am I hurting? I'm not hurting anyone. NO ONE—especially not God. The love I feel for God and the love I feel God has for me is AMAZING! My relationship with God is AMAZING! Who can argue with that?! If you are someone who doesn't agree, don't be angry that I feel the way I do. Like I said, this is something God put in my heart, and it's not going anywhere.

When the multiple sclerosis began to change my life, it began to change the lives of my family as well. The normal life that we had became pretty much nonexistent. One night, Dan was working late. The kids were fighting in the basement, that normal still existed. I was in the kitchen making mac and cheese. Carrying the pot to the sink to drain the noodles, some water spilled on the floor. I just fell next to the spilled water and began to cry.

"This isn't fair, God. Zac and Shaina don't have a normal mom. They have more responsibilities because of the MS. They can't do normal things with their

mom. *Their mom uses a wheelchair. Dan doesn't have a normal wife. He's the one who does the cooking and cleaning. My family does NOT have a normal life.*"

As I was in the midst of feeling sorry for myself, God interrupted my pity party and gave me a revelation that we could handle this. Zac and Shaina came running upstairs to see what had happened. I told them, "God said we could handle the MS. God must think we are really strong. God is NEVER wrong. Let's make God proud of us. We can handle this." I got up from the floor, dried my tears, and finished making the mac and cheese. I felt so much better.

Shaina came home from school the next day (I think she was in 6th grade). I can still see her walking through the door and up the steps into the kitchen. Even before saying hello, she looked at me and with all seriousness and said, "Mom, I will always do what you ask without complaining, except if I'm in a really bad mood."

I couldn't help but smile. I knew she had been thinking about what was said the night before at school that day. Shaina kept her word. Of course, being a girl, the older she gets, the bad mood comes A LOT more often. I never really felt sorry for my family again, and they don't feel sorry for me either. This is our life. Dan used to say this was our normal (of course, he also said I was never normal). Whatever. God is right though, we can handle this.

Even though Zac and Shaina can handle this, it's important to me that they have good memories. I don't want my kids just to remember how hard their life was. It is true that they have more responsibilities. At the beginning, it was only simple (simple, yet annoying) things that I was finding difficult to do. "Could you please run upstairs and get something, run down stairs and get something, carry this, pick up that." Though I always tried to make sure Zac and Shaina knew I appreciated what they did for me (hope I did), as it became more than doing simple things, saying thank you no longer felt enough. A strong desire developed that I needed to show Zac and Shaina my appreciation. I came up with an idea to either buy them something or pay them. Not anything big and not because I have to, because I want to. Dan may not be in total agreement— he did NOT have the same desire—but this is about how I feel. I'm sure some will say I'm bribing them. I'm not. ALL RIGHT, I did bribe them a few times. Don't judge. Sometimes things just need to get done. You got to do what you got to do. It's more that I want to reward them for good behavior. Don't misunderstand, I'm not talking about doing normal chores. I personally think its good, GREAT for kids to have chores to teach them responsibility. What I'm talking about is when Zac and Shaina do things that I used to do and no longer do, things I SHOULD be doing but don't because of the multiple sclerosis.

When I stopped driving, I started needing someone to drive me and my wheelchair. Zac drives me to do errands. Being my chauffeur has kind of become his job. I'm sure there are many times that Zac would rather be making plans with his friends but he can't because he needs to drive me somewhere. Shaina helps with the wash and ironing. Our laundry room is in the basement. Steps and no bathroom are not a good combination for me. The wash and ironing has kind of become Shaina's job. I remember one day when Zac was taking me to the mall, and I asked Shaina twice if she wanted to go. She said no. Walking out the door, I glanced downstairs and saw my young daughter ironing. Shaina was choosing to stay home so she could get the wash and ironing done. At that moment I felt this incredible love for my daughter. At the same time, I knew that if I didn't reward her, I'd feel like the wicked stepmother. Does it matter that I work part time at Express Clothing and maybe there was something she wanted? NO, it didn't matter to me. I didn't feel like the wicked stepmother.

Rewarding Zac and Shaina helps ME feel so much better about this yucky situation. And the kids have ABSOLUTELY no problem with it. Shaina has done quite well in the clothes department. I've had a few people tell me how having a sick parent made their childhood so difficult. Hearing stories like that always make me sad. I feel sad for them. I also feel sad for me. All it does is remind me that I'm in the same position of doing that to my kids. I don't want to do that to my kids. Those are not memories I want for Zac and Shaina. So, yes, I love my rewarding idea. Though I will say that if the good behavior or a good attitude happens to be absent, the strong desire is absent also.

If you are in a similar situation, I'm not telling you that you have to reward your kids or that you should feel guilty if you don't. I just wanted to share what helps me and how I was trying to help Zac and Shaina find some good in this bad. I don't want my kids to resent me. More importantly, I don't want my kids to resent God because they had to grow up with a mom who had a disease. God gave us free will and life is full of choices. We make choices every day. One choice I choose to make is to have a positive attitude about the multiple sclerosis. It takes work. I don't always succeed. But I know when I AM happy and have a positive attitude, I feel better physically and my family is much happier. Sure, I have bad days when it's hard to smile and be positive. 98% of the time, it has nothing to do with multiple sclerosis. Being a mom of teenagers is hard. Being a wife can be really hard. I don't handle things the way I should a lot. The devil knows my weakness (as does Zac) and I find it doesn't help that I have just a tiny issue with repeating. I figure that comes from the fact my family never seem to listen to me. Dan and Shaina have even said to me numerous times, "What did you just say? I totally was not listening." Oh, there are so many moments I need more prayer for being a mom (or wife) than for multiple sclerosis.

Every day your kids learn from you. They watch how you live your life. They watch how you handle things. What would I be teaching Zac and Shaina if I blamed God, cried, or was depressed all the time? How would that help them on their walk with God? Your attitude affects everything about your life. Your attitude affects everyone in your life. Sometimes it IS hard to be happy, no one can make you be happy, but a negative attitude will make a situation so much worse. Having a positive attitude doesn't mean we have to like our situation. Being positive will help you endure it—God's Grace will get you through it. With God's help, you will find happiness. For a long time I thought having a positive attitude meant I had to accept multiple sclerosis for my life. I thought it meant giving up on being healed. But no, being positive means I want to be happy and I want my family to be happy while waiting for God to heal me. I don't have to give up on anything.

You may not be able to change your situation, but you can change your attitude. Being happy is a way better way to live. As a parent, you are the most important teacher your kids will ever have. Whatever life brings, good or bad, teach your kids about God. Especially in hard times, teach your kids that faith in God brings you strength. When your prayers aren't answered the way you want, teach your kids to never stop praying. Show them you don't ever give up on God. That is what I want Zac and Shaina to remember. I never gave up on God. That is a memory they can tell anyone.

Your life is a gift. If your life isn't turning out the way you thought it should, don't waste your life, the gift God gave you, with feelings of bitterness or self-pity. Those feelings will hurt you. I know I already talked about how important it is to have a positive attitude, but just go with me here. When those feelings turn into words, it will do more than just hurt you. Proverbs 8:21 says, "Death and life are in the power of the tongue; and they that love it shall eat the fruit thereof." The Message is a bit more direct: "Words kill, words give life, they're either poison or fruit—you choose."

My point here is that the words we say are SO important and its OUR choice what we say—key word being 'OUR'. James 3:6 tells us the tongue is a restless evil full of deadly poison. We can do so much damage with our words, in more ways than one. Friends, when we turn negative feelings into words, when we whine and complain about our life—or about anything for that matter—besides poisoning your future (WHICH YOU WILL DO) and annoying your family and driving your friends away (WHICH YOU WILL DO), you are agreeing with the devil. I'm sure you've heard the saying: Don't talk the problem; talk the answer. Great advice, but I have another one for ya: Stop agreeing with the devil; start agreeing with God.

I'll be honest, there are times when agreeing with God is the last thing on my mind. There have been times when I've even yelled, "I AM SO WEAK!" That is NOT agreeing with God. Who cares how weak I feel? Okay, maybe I do care, but STILL, God says let the weak say I am strong. I should be yelling, "I AM SO STRONG!" I say to myself all the time, "Do not be moved by what you feel, only be moved by the word of God." And the word of God says in Isaiah 4:29 that "God gives strength to the weary and increases the power of the weak." Why is it so hard to take advice from God? Seriously, I should be yelling, "I AM SO STRONG!"

There are so many reasons why we should be in God's word. The Bible says in Mark 4:4 that "man shall not live by bread alone, but by every word that comes out of the mouth of God." We need to be in God's word to live. God's words are life and health. I have come to realize that this one book is key to everything in this world. The Bible has verses that will encourage you, give you direction, teach you, inspire you, comfort you, give you hope, correct you, and confuse you (just kidding. No, not really. Deuteronomy 29:29 says the secret things belong to the Lord our God… a good verse to keep handy). The Bible is full of promises from God. The Bible is full of God. "In the beginning was the word, and the word was with God, and the word was God" (John 1:1). The Bible IS God.

I want to share a few of my favorite Bible verses:

Psalm 118:24: "This is the day the Lord has made, let us rejoice and be glad in it." The Bible doesn't say tomorrow or when my life gets better or even when I'm healed. The Bible says THIS is the day. Today is the day.

Isaiah 41:10: "So do not fear for I am with you, do not be dismayed for I am your God. I will strengthen you and help you, I will uphold you with my righteous right hand."

Psalm 18:1: "I love you O Lord, my strength." God is my strength, literally. This trial does drain me, but the joy of the Lord strengthens me (Nehemiah 8:10).

Matthew 9:22, Mark 5:34: "Jesus turned and saw her. 'Take heart, daughter.' He said, 'Your faith has healed you.' And the woman was healed from that moment. 'Daughter, your faith has healed you. Go in peace and be freed from your suffering.'" I love to close my eyes and imagine Jesus saying this to me.

Psalm 103:2-3: "Praise the Lord, O my soul and forget not all his benefits, who forgives all your sins and heals all your diseases." Healing is a benefit. God will heal just as he will forgive sins—SAME SENTENCE.

1 John 4:4: "You dear children, are from God and have overcome them, because the one who is in you is greater than the one who is in the world." The devil may be in this world, but I have God in me, and God is WAY stronger than the devil.

*Hebrews 13:8: "Jesus Christ is the same yesterday, today, and forever." By read-
ing the gospels, we get to know Jesus, and we see that when Jesus walked the
earth he healed everyone. He didn't say to some, "I'm not going to heal you, it's
my plan for you to be sick and suffer." God didn't say it was His plan for them
to be used this way. NO, Jesus healed EVERYONE of all manner of sickness
and all manner of disease. Colossians 1:15 tells us that Jesus is the image of the
invisible God. And this verse says that Jesus is the same today as he was then.
Why, then, is it so hard for people to believe that God will heal today on this
earth? I'm claiming my promise. I have nothing to lose and everything to gain.*

*Romans 12:12: "Be joyful in hope, patient in affliction, faithful in prayer."
This verse has become my MS verse. This verse reminds me how I should live
my life with this disease. We, as Christians, have hope, because we have God.
I have hope for a miracle, and that makes me happy. I am joyful in hope. And
about being patient in affliction, IT'S HARD. Especially when God's timing
isn't our timing. It's good for me to be reminded to be patient. AND it's good
to be reminded to be faithful in prayer. Prayer needs to be a priority. I feel that
successful living with multiple sclerosis is to be happy, be patient, and to pray.*

*Matthew 22:37: "Love the Lord your God with all your heart and with all
your soul and with all your mind." I do love God with all my heart, soul, and
mind. I've loved God my whole life. But there were times I doubted God's goodness and questioned his love for me. I questioned the MS. I questioned, "Why
me?" Yet I always found that questioning God never made me feel any better.
Questioning God, especially questioning His love, only made me feel worse. I
no longer question God about His love for me. I know how much God loves
me. Although I no longer doubt God's goodness or love, that doesn't mean that
struggles are not there. I do, in times of frustration, often question God and his
timing. I don't want MS anymore. I want to be a normal mom and a normal
wife. I want to do normal things. Sometimes I just feel like screaming, "GOD,
TAKE THIS AWAY!" I will say that I'm learning to give God my struggles and
frustrations. This sickness does get me down, some days more than others. But
it doesn't keep me down—emotionally, physically, or spiritually. When I fall to
my knees and cry to God, I never stay there. I do eventually get up and tell God
how much I love him.*

2 Corinthians 5:7: "We live by faith, not by sight." The Bible has taught me so much about faith. I learned that faith is believing without seeing. There are many people who think that they need to see a miracle for their faith to be strengthened. Faith doesn't work that way. Faith is sticking with God and his Word no matter WHAT happens in life. Hebrews 11:1 says, "Now faith is being sure of what we hope for and certain of what we do not see." When we don't see what we want and believe anyway, that's the faith God wants us to have. That's the faith I want to have. In Romans 4, we read about Abraham's faith. The Bible says that without weakening in his faith, Abraham faced the fact that his body was as good as dead and Sarah's womb was also dead. "Yet he did not waiver through unbelief regarding the promise of God, but was strengthened in his faith and gave glory to God" (Romans 4:20). Abraham didn't waver, he never looked at the situation or how hopeless it seemed. Abraham kept his eyes on the promise. Against all hope, in hope Abraham believed and became the father of many nations. I don't think faith makes God work in your life, I believe faith allows God to work in your life. Abraham kept his faith and God did work in his life. I'm not denying that MS is real in my life, but so is God, and nothing is impossible for God (Luke 1:37). One might say that there being no cure for MS is no hope. However, against all hope, I will keep believing. I need to be sure of what I hope for and certain of what I do not see, because "everything is possible for him who believes" (Mark 9:23).

Lastly, I want to share Psalm 27:13 with you. This verse means the most to me. "I am still confident of this—that I will see the goodness of the Lord in the land of the living." One day, I received a note in the mail that said God had given this person a verse for me. It was THIS verse. I was so excited. God had given me that same verse years ago with the thought that healing is goodness. I don't know who sent that note to me; it wasn't signed. I still have it tucked in my Bible. After receiving that note, I knew that I was going to be healed on Earth.

God impressed on my heart that I needed to stop looking at what's wrong in my life. I needed to find the good in my life and hold on to it—so I did. I found many good things. My husband, Dan, is good in my life. I don't know when God plans on healing me. Zac and Shaina will grow up, get married, have their own families, in that order, and I'm fairly certain they will move

*out someday. But this is Dan's life, and he's not going anywhere. That is what
I tell him.*

*One morning as I was making my way down the stairs, I saw Dan in the din-
ing room. I couldn't help but sit right where I was on the step and look at him.
As I was thinking how much I loved him (I must have had a good night), God
reminded me that I'm not the only one with multiple sclerosis. Dan has it too.
No, he's not affected physically (maybe with his back—he does carry me if it is
needed), but his life is affected. When a man and a women get married, when
they make vows to each other, the two become one. When those vows are honored, what affects one will affect the other. Dan's life is affected in SO MANY
WAYS. I'm quite positive having a wife with multiple sclerosis was NOT what
Dan planned for his life. I have opportunities to be a witness for God, but so
does Dan. People are watching him too, especially our kids. Dan is being a
witness for God by honoring his wedding vows. He loves me in sickness and in
health; in good times and in bad times.*

*He is also being a witness by how he handles this disease. Dan has many days
that he gets sick and tired. Dan has many days he gets frustrated with the
multiple sclerosis and it's obvious that he's working hard at having a positive
attitude. Yet Dan is good to me. I feel blessed and thankful that I have Dan on
this journey with me. HOWEVER, I'm not going to tell you that he's perfect,
because he's not. I am not going to tell you that we have a perfect marriage, because we don't. He might say that I have a slight problem with always needing
to be right (whatever). I might say that he has a slight problem with moodiness
(HE DOES).*

*Seriously, there have been some big, huge, gigantic, massive, enormous issues
in our marriage that we had to get through. The loving in good and bad times
SOOOOOOOOOOOOOO goes both ways. We've had small issues. Good grief,
we STILL have issues. He is a man. Did I just say that? I think I did. Now,
this would be a small issue, but I had an idea of how a furniture store could
sell more furniture, or at least more bedroom furniture. If they threw socks on
the floor and hung clothes over the bedposts, a man would see it and think,
*That would work, *and it would help the woman visualize the furniture in
her home. Honestly, marriage is hard work with or without a trial. The devil*

must work overtime in marriages. Look around—it has to be true. If you are married or are getting married, put your armor on and KEEP IT ON. If not now, you WILL need it later. Anyway, I do feel like it was God's plan for us to be together because, really, we're good together. Whether Dan admits it or not, he needs me as much as I need him. Okay, not quite as much and maybe not in the same way, but he still needs me. I tell him that too. My kids are also a very good thing in my life. So are my family, my friends, my church, my house, my makeup, and my couch. I even found something good with the multiple sclerosis (could be more about finding good in the bad) besides getting the best parking. I get to take naps. Dan tells me to go rest a lot. Forget the reason why I need the naps. I GET TO TAKE NAPS. What woman in this world wouldn't love to hear her husband tell her that she should go rest and he'll get dinner. Why the naps are needed is TOTALLY out of my mind.

There is something else that I do find to be good; I always have an 'in' to talk about God. One time, I was getting my nails done, and this young woman who was sitting next to me asked why I was in the wheelchair. I told her I had multiple sclerosis. She then asked what that was. I told her. She looks at me and said, "That sucks." I almost started laughing—actually, I think I did. What a great way to describe multiple sclerosis. Sorry, Mom (she hates that word). I told this young woman that yes, it does suck (again, sorry Mom). And then I told her how God gets me through every day. That was the end of our conversation. Just maybe, if she ever has a hard time in her life, she'll remember the woman in the wheelchair getting her nails done. Multiple sclerosis has given me many chances to talk about God. I can't even tell you how many great God conversations I've had getting my nails done. The BEST thing in my life for sure is my relationship with Jesus Christ. Anyone can have that be their best. Life on Earth is temporary; heaven is for eternity. The Bible says that the trials we have, the pain and suffering, and the devil's attacks are not going to be in heaven with us. The devil is not going to be in heaven with us. Now that's something really good to hold onto.

What I want to tell you is to not to wait until you have a trial before you spend time in God's word—do it now. If you have a trial, find out what God says about your situation. Write those verses down. Claim those verses every day. Get them in your head, get them in your heart and agree with God. Read your

Bible and sharpen your sword. It's hard to fight a lion with a dull sword. Spend time in prayer. The Bible says to pray continually (1 Thessalonians 5:17). Talk to God like he's right there with you, because he is. And don't just talk, listen for his voice. We can talk to God in our thoughts, and we can talk to God out loud. Either way works. Personally, I love to have conversations with God out loud. YEP, Zac and Shaina are totally convinced I talk to myself. It's okay though, when I talk to myself (because I do), I tell them I'm talking to God. It's not a total lie, God IS listening. And always remember to spend time praising God. Praise God for who God is, not just for what God does. I think many times, people get caught up in their lives, trials or no trials, and they get selfish. They forget that life is about God. The thing is, life isn't about us or what God can do for us, life is about God and what we can do for him, what we become IN him. We need to get the focus off ourselves and focus on God.

One morning, I was having a hard time walking. I fell to my knees and started to cry, which seems to be a pattern for me. The devil was working on me and was winning this battle. I had the radio on and a song started playing that I never heard before. Suddenly the tears stopped and I was lifting my hands, praising God. The focus was no longer on me. I had an awesome experience with God. Amazing things happen when you praise God. HE SHOWS UP. Attitudes change and the devil loses.

What I believe God wants to tell you to keep your eyes on him. If your life isn't turning out as you had planned, if you think he's not listening to your prayers, TRUST HIM. God does hear you. God loves you and will ALWAYS be with you.

Multiple sclerosis is a small trial. There are many and MUCH harder trials that people go through. I was getting my nails done (Okay, I like getting manicures. Besides feeling good when my nails look nice, manicures are WAY cheaper than therapy.) and I started talking to this lady next to me. I was telling this woman how God gets me through my days with multiple sclerosis. All of a sudden, she looks at me and says, "I can't believe I'm going to tell you this" and proceeds to tell me about her son who was dying of liver cancer. For an instant, I felt SO inadequate. I didn't know what to say. I was humbled. My trial is NOTHING compared to hers. After I left, I couldn't stop thinking about that lady or the conversation we had. I couldn't stop thinking how all I did was share with her how God helps me live with my trial. Then I realized something. Our trials and our situations are way different, but our God is the same.

There was a time when I would pray, "God, if you'll heal me, I'll go on Oprah, and tell everyone how awesome you are. I'll show them that miracles really do happen." And I will still do that (maybe). Why do I need to be healed before I tell anyone how awesome God is. Isn't he a good God now? Oh yes, he's a good God now. And I'm not going to wait until I'm healed before I tell anyone how awesome God is. God is an AWESOME God.

Sometimes things happen in life that make it hard to see beyond our pain. Who am I kidding? A LOT of things happen that make it hard to see beyond our pain. Don't be angry at God. Don't run away from God. Run to him. Psalm 105:4 says, "Seek the Lord and his strength, seek his presence continually." Seek the Lord, seek his strength. There is sadness in this life. Things happen that will bring unbelievable sadness. And yes, things happen that bring disappointment. We will be sad. I want to encourage you not to stay there. God understands your need to be there. Just don't stay there. Give God your sadness. God will give you the strength you need to get through it.

Multiple sclerosis was not what I had planned for my life. But I'm not going to waste time feeling sorry for myself. I have a choice to make and I choose to be happy. I'm not a Christian with a perfect life. I have struggles every day in MANY areas. As a person, I'm far from perfect. I have a lot to learn. My husband and kids would be quick to agree. But I have no doubt of what God has done in my life. I have no doubt of what my faith has done for my life. And I know what having a relationship with Jesus Christ means to me. God is my life. And God helps me live every day with this disease. If you are having struggles in your life, give God a chance. Stay or get an attitude of faith. Let God have an opportunity to work in your life. Because he will if you let him. I will always believe in my miracle, BUT if I die tomorrow—I'M NOT GOING TO—but if I did, I wouldn't want people to say, "That poor girl believed in her healing on Earth, and God never healed her." For one thing, don't feel bad for me if I died. I'd be healed in heaven with God. And another thing, don't ever feel bad that I believed in my healing on Earth. My life is lived having faith in God.

That faith gives me hope. That hope makes me happy. I'm HAPPY. Nothing more will need to be said.

I want to leave you with this, get excited about God and get excited about your life, whatever your situation is. When you get excited about God, you will be excited about your life. I know it works; it worked for me. I can't wait to see what else God has planned—maybe I should get some nerve pills. And more importantly, I want to leave you with this. What do people see when they look at you? You may be the only Jesus that someone ever sees. I have heard people say that's pressure. That's not pressure. That, my friend, is a privilege.

I hope I've encouraged you in some way. Thanks for listening.

It's been years since I wrote that speech. Every time I read it, I'm reminded of the special place I was with God at that time in my life. I'm reminded that my trial, my life, is NOTHING compared to others'. Though there have been changes since that speech was written, my purpose and prayer for this speech is still the same—to encourage in some way and see that when life doesn't turn out the way we plan, we need to put and keep our eyes on God. That being said, about the changes, keep reading.

Chapter 3

Living Life, Loving God

I live life loving God. My life seemed to be going as planned until symptoms of this dreaded disease showed up and changed my life and that of my family. But I was determined to have a smile on my face, and with God that was possible. I always did my best to smile. Of course, having Dan, Zac, and Shaina, a nice house, and an excuse to stay in bed and take naps didn't hurt either. Due to health changes, we moved from where we had lived for 17 years. The whole house situation had more 'WOW' stories than I ever thought possible. I really was at a great place with God. BUT, the way I felt about God at that time was NOTHING compared to the way I feel about God presently. I have always felt God loves me and have believed that He does not desire me to live with this disease, but I believed that someday God would heal me—someday.

I had been working on this book for while when a friend shared with me what God had put in her heart. She ordered a teaching by a TV evangelist, and we, along with another friend, started a Bible study that began to renew my mind. I began to see healing differently. My love for God was taken to a whole new level. A few days after our Monday morning Bible study, I felt the need to get up and walk, so I got up and walked with no assistance. I felt so much excitement; it had been years since the last time that happened, but when God told me, "Man says there is no cure, I say there is a cure, and his name is Jesus Christ," my someday changed to THIS day.

I requested a King James Bible for Christmas that year. I know people struggle with this version, my family included. They totally questioned my gift idea. Despite the numerous questions, Zac bought me one anyway. I can't say it was my favorite gift because that would not be fair (but it was). I will say that it became my favorite translation. I discovered that the more I read, the more God's word became alive. I did not mark up this Bible, I wanted each verse to be as if I were reading it for the first time. Instead, I bought index cards and filled them with the verses that became alive to me. I had such a hunger for God—a hunger that only His word could fill. My mind was renewing; I was becoming transformed.

Soon after, the infusions for my multiple sclerosis were stopped. Informing my kids and my parents that I'd stopped the medicine and believed in my healing today rather than later and telling my friends where the infusion took place that I was stopping led to more God stories. NO, I am NOT telling anyone to quit taking medicine. God put doctors on this earth, and if a cure did become available in the form of medicine, I would be all over that baby. But there is NO medical cure for MS, and it was put in my heart a long time ago that it would not be modern medicine that would heal me.

Anyway, I had written in detail several God stories that took place, but unfortunately, those pages cannot be found! I remember writing about feeling lonely and feeling that a couple of friends gave up believing in my healing because it was taking so long. I remember writing about me and Dan going to see his dad at the nursing home and how I saw God encouraging me as I walked to Dad's room. I remember writing about being empty-nesters and that Dan could make a hamburger dish he called Wednesday Night Surprise any night of the week (the kids were NOT a fan of this particular food dish). I wrote about a time when Dan rushed into the house because he was sure that I'd fallen, but it was just me singing LOUDLY to praise music! So much was written. Oh well!

I was very fortunate and very grateful to have no symptoms of multiple sclerosis during Zac and Shaina's younger years. I smile and thank God for the memories. Talking to Dan about all the memories one day, I could not stop laughing at remembering a time when I had taken the kids to a local Christian bookstore to see some novelty. I believe Shaina was around 3, and as we got in the car afterward, I noticed that her pockets were bulging. When I questioned her, she began to cry. I came to discover that my daughter had a pocketful of those small red Bibles. I had her march right back and return them and say she was sorry. My daughter was a thief, and my son an innocent bystander. I remember Zac sitting in the car so quietly. He was probably relieved that he wasn't the one in trouble. I did buy one for each of them—come on, THEY WERE BIBLES! Does that memory ever bring laughter and a smile to my heart. Oh yes, how fortunate and grateful I am that I was able to be a mom who loved them, loved their father, and so loved life.

Looking back, I realize how blessed I was and am—growing up as I did, my mom and dad, my sisters, the love felt, all the happy memories. In fact, I had a dear uncle comment on how blessed I am to have my mom and both my sisters live within 15 minutes of me. And I will comment that we also are very close emotionally, including the brother-in-laws.

I do question—why my story? There are way worse journeys than mine. Many disturbing stories, unnecessary deaths, young dying, unheard-of diseases, struggling marriages—so many journeys are way worse and there are journeys way better than mine! Seriously God, why mine? WHY ME? Is it because we need to hear a good testimony? It seems we always hear about something bad or painful that was endured. We live in a broken world with evil happening every day, and it is helpful to hear how a person got through a bad situation! Maybe this book has something to do with people needing GOOD stories. I often close my eyes and remind myself how good I have it. God reminds me how good I have it a lot. Is that why I need to tell my story? I did not nor do I presently live an abundant life, but I do live a blessed life! Maybe that's why God wants me to write this book, to share the GOOD on my journey. Book upon books are written without a mention of God. This world needs to hear a testimony about how advice was taken and how someone learned from the Bible—someone who learned from GOD, NOT SATAN.

I remember so vividly telling God one morning that I was being used for Him in the wheelchair at the mall (I worked in a mall). God politely informed me that that was about ME, not Him. Really? That shocked me—

my positive attitude and smile is about me? I thought it was for God! People who know me know that it's because of God that I smile. God told me that that was true, but I am surrounded by people who DON'T know me or my story. A person may say, "That girl in the wheelchair has such a good attitude," and leave it at that. I would get the glory, not God. Walking normally, strangers wouldn't know I was healed.

Oh good grief, you're right, God, my positive attitude and smile ARE about me. I'm AT A MALL. I'M SO SORRY, GOD!

As I was taking a break from writing and eating my waffle, a thought came to me that I'm going to become the woman healed of multiple sclerosis. People talk and word will get around that I was the one in the wheelchair, the girl with the positive attitude, the one healed from an incurable disease. The only explanation could be God. The only explanation WILL be God.

Years and years ago, while sitting on the front steps of our previous home watching my husband pull weeds, a thought came to me that the devil is a like a weed. I believed that thought was a great analogy for Satan. Weeds are pulled but always come back. Just like evil, you rebuke but the devil always comes back. Some weeds appear as flowers. We had a purple flower in our grass that I found to be nice looking. It could be that I love that shade of purple, but whatever, Dan informed me that was a weed and it had to go. Bummer, there goes most of our yard—oh well. Isn't that just like the devil to make sin appear appealing. Come on people, it's STILL SIN! The devil is such a weed.

Another thought that came to me years ago is that Jesus is the softer side of God. Read the gospels and see if you don't feel the same way. Years and more years ago, my sister shared something with me that was way too cute not to share with you. My young nephew had wanted a glass of water with his meal and my sister told him that he couldn't have water until he finished drinking his milk. His reply still makes me laugh. He told his mom that that was fine—he would just drink his tears. Cute, huh?

Most mornings, the only thing on my mind is how good the bed feels. I love bedtime. I love sleeping. Insomnia stinks. I found prayer to be a good in that bad. I crawl in bed, put on my earphones and fall asleep listening to various God teachings on my iPod. That brings a memory to my mind. When Zac was little, I'd have to put a cassette tape of a sermon in his Fisher Price player to help him fall asleep. That brings another memory to mind of me dancing like a crazy woman to his favorite song before bedtime prayers. We always listened to one song before bedtime prayers.

Anyway, most Christians, as do I, believe that when we die, we are immediately with God. Jesus told the thief on the cross that today—TODAY—he would be with him in paradise. Then again, the Bible also refers to death as falling asleep, and those asleep will wake up when Jesus comes back. So, which is it? RHONDA, IT DOESN'T MATTER! YOU'RE WITH ME!

I love to go and watch movies. Some theaters even have reclining seats. I saw the movie "The Shack" and though horrifying events took place, and God or the Trinity may have not been portrayed the same as a person imagines, God met the main character where he was. I totally enjoyed this movie. I felt it portrayed God in such a loving way, as was Jesus and the Holy Spirit. Many people found fault with it, but I feel many are missing the boat here. I happen to be excited to see this movie again. I still think about it. I'm not thinking about the sad things that happened, I'm thinking about God's love and how God cares and meets you where you are. We should not be criticizing such movies but wanting more of them. It may get a person to search the Bible and see what the Bible says; it might open a door and be exactly what they need.

Speaking of movies, in the movie 'Passion of the Christ', a magnificent scene happens immediately after Jesus dies. They show the devil angry. Many people probably missed that scene. I know my mom did (her eyes were still closed after all of the bloody scenes). I saw it, understood it, and loved it.

I was sitting in church one Sunday and listening to the piano and guitar play so beautifully during collection with my eyes closed. I felt God's presence enjoying it with me. I opened my eyes and saw empty pews and thought, *Why are the pews not full, how sad the pews aren't full.* All I could think was, *What is wrong with you people?* It was like seeing empty seats at a Christian movie. *WHAT IS WRONG WITH YOU PEOPLE?* There are so many hurting people, so many hurting children of God. The devil is so running wild. Those who are dear to me, the WORLD needs to see GOD run wild! RUN, GOD, RUN! God told Dan that I needed to write a book. So, I'm writing a book. I happen to be excited to see where this plan leads. Here's a thought, LET'S FIND OUT TOGETHER!

Chapter 4

God's Word is Alive

I knew this would be an important chapter, but I had NO idea how important it would be for me. I was thinking this chapter was to be verses God spoke to me from the King James, New International, and the Message versions of the Bible, side by side. Different translations speak to people differently—everyone has their favorite. The chapter was even started that way. However, not knowing where to begin or end because of all the verses made me feel overwhelmed, I found myself playing computer games instead of writing. Fun, yes! Addictive, yes! Productive, not so much!

One morning, while playing spider solitaire, a sudden and out-of-the-blue thought came to me about how this chapter should be written. I took my index cards and combined the verses into one paragraph.

When I read it to Dan, his only comment was: "That's a lot of verses."

I think it bored him. Feeling perplexed AND overwhelmed, I found myself once again playing games instead of writing. A week or so later, more sudden and out-of-the-blue thoughts on how this chapter should be written came to me. I took the continuous thought from God, personalized the verses and began to arrange them in a way that I felt God wanted me to hear them. God was helping me write a prescription that would become my medicine—that would become my cure!

Am I ever excited, the butterflies in my stomach are enormous. But why was I finding the prescription difficult to write, though? God put the idea in my head, right? It has been said to find a verse or verses in the Bible that apply to your situation, write them down, and say them every day. Nothing new, I've done that. People pull verses all the time. It has been said to personalize verses. All right, that was something more new, but I understood the need to claim the verse for your own. So why was the prescription difficult to write? Maybe it wasn't God who put the prescription idea in my head.

Then, one day, while reading the great big mountain of words, "Seek and ye shall find" came to my heart. I did seek. I did find. I found Jesus in a way He wasn't seen before. God told me that Jesus is the cure. Jesus is the word. The word is my cure. It WAS God. I'm going to see my healing—on THIS earth! I feel overwhelmed by God's love. This time, feeling overwhelmed was incredible.

I shared with my husband all that had transpired. Dan asked what I thought would happen next. I told him that I didn't know but believed with all my heart that complete healing would be seen. It probably would have been best to leave the completely healed part out until the prescription was finished because Dan keeps bugging me that I need to be done working on it and begin taking it ASAP. I do agree, this medicine should be finished. He's right—who wouldn't start taking a medicine that would heal them as soon as possible? This medicine is not as quick as taking a pill, it's long and many may find it boring. I'm pretty sure if told this medicine would bring healing to an incurable disease you had, the word 'boring' would not be in your vocabulary. Many may have struggles and this medicine may not make sense.

Thinking about struggles some may have, this was put in my heart: "Let me assure you—this is not replacing the Bible. This is merely a prescription."

Really? Thanks God! Couldn't have said it better myself. About it not making sense, this is my personal medicine—verses that became alive to me, words God wants me to hear, words I NEED to hear and say daily—it makes sense to me. Where the verses are found is not included with the prescription. This is not a how-to book. It is not about how to receive a miracle or what verses you need to receive a miracle. This book is about my journey. Whatever your journey, God has words for you. Seek and find your own words. Find God for yourself. Let God speak through verses that become alive to YOU!

The plan is to be done writing and concentrate on my healing and God's amazing love. So like the infusion treatment for MS, I'm going to sit in a comfy chair and let the medicine flow through my body.

My Prescription...

NOPE, this is not my prescription.

Six months later and I'm still working on it. WHAT? But I was all set to begin taking it. REALLY? I was all set to concentrate on healing and God's love. IT'S NOT DONE? Looks like another changed plan. That's too bad, I liked that plan. It feels as though I'm a scientist working on a cure. This medicine is only for me, but hey, it's exciting. Due to lack of certain brain cells along with my husband insisting I have symptoms of some sort of an obsessive compulsive disorder, feeling like a scientist is as close as I'm going to get to that 'as if'. I'm not making light of OCD, it is another terrible disease, but I agree to some sort of something. I've always had my suspicions. It was just never an issue.

I remember writing my speech and now the prescription, and things need to be perfect. Not perfect to the world, but perfect to me. Looking back, there was a time in particular where perfection became an issue.

Shaina has no 1-year photo. That is no big deal, but it does prove my obsession with perfection. Zac wore a sailor outfit for his photos, and I thought that since our kids were close in age, Shaina should also wear a sailor outfit for her photos, and being a girl, a sailor dress would be perfect. When she turned 1, couldn't find a sailor dress anywhere. So Shaina has no 1-year photos, she probably always wondered why she doesn't have 1-year photos when her brother has such cute professional photos. Sorry, Shaina. It was your mother's obsession with perfection. I still feel bad about it.

Okay, I just asked Shaina if I could read her something I had written, She said she didn't want to hear it, the tears shed while reading what was written to Dan, the regret felt that Shaina had no 1-year picture...all GONE. Once again, a moment of silence is needed to long for middle school years. Shhhh, I just need a moment. Shaina was informed that I'd be writing about this. Permission was granted.

Anyway, my need for perfection can easily turn into a problem, and unfortunately, God isn't the only one who knows about my issue with perfection. It took a while to figure out that the devil was messing with me regarding the prescription. The devil knows changes will continue to be made if felt God wants something changed, and if I say this is the medicine I took, it has to be EXACTLY the medicine I took. And here I was under the impression that writing a book would be easier than speaking. It's NOT! The good in this apparent bad is all the time spent with God. Looks like the joke is on the devil because I'm having LOTS of God time.

While showering one morning, I heard, "The devil is fighting dirty," thinking God was referring to my health, it didn't bother me. I can handle my health. That's about ME, and besides, I have the word to back up my feelings on healing. Boy, was I wrong! A day that next week, my husband had given me his phone before having a medical procedure, and for no reason, I looked at Dan's phone and noticed a number twice. Dan uses his phone for work, so the same number more than once would be common. Why was I so bothered by this? True we've had and still have trials in our marriage, and MS is no help, but I have been with Dan for over half my life. We have children, we have history, we have memories. Regardless of any past or present trial, I want to grow old with this man. Thoughts are how God speaks to me. God has spoken to me for years through thoughts. I DON'T KNOW WHAT TO DO WITH THIS! Why is this happening? I do NOT want this!

A couple days after sharing the phone incident with Dan, it became clear why this was happening. I will never forget being downstairs and telling Dan that "The cares of the world choke the word," kept coming to me. I care about my marriage. I care about Dan. I have been planting healing verses. I have been planting God. Dan and our marriage have become the cares of my world. Satan was trying to take the word out of my heart. The devil knows what the word can do and the power that's in it. God's glory would be seen with my healing and the word would be verified. It all makes sense—the devil wants to distract me. The devil doesn't want me healed. It was said in my speech that the devil's number one place to attack is marriage.

I see times when sin tried to creep into my life; I see times when sin DID creep into my life. But I also see times when God protected me from sin. And God didn't have to creep. Of course the devil attacks my marriage—I should be ENCOURAGED! The Bible tells us that the thief is only here to kill, steal, and destroy. God calls the devil a THIEF! A thief takes that which belongs to you, right? Healing belongs to ME! It all makes sense.

Satan can't hurt God directly but hurts God by hurting His children. Attacking a marriage is a two-for-one. Actually, it's a more-for-one, since kids, parents, family, and friends can all be affected. I diligently sought God. I believe in my healing. I'm excited to verify the word. Oh my gosh, yes. It's so clear why this is happening. Satan does NOT want me to be healed.

Here, months later, no one knows about the toll MS or believing for my healing has taken on my marriage, or that the prescription isn't finished and I haven't been taking the medicine as intended. Though our kids are aware of much, even they don't know that (well, okay, I did share some of what's going on with a few close friends). I have seen ways evil has been trying to destroy my marriage for years. It's easy to think the devil is working not only in my mind but my husband's. True, there are marriages that survive, couples who honor their vows and stay together through trials of many sorts. Yes, marriage is difficult and when a trial of any sort IS added—ouch! I'm well aware of what this disease and believing in my healing is doing to my marriage. Oh my gosh, I'm SO aware!

The time it is taking to write this book really does suck. The MS sucks. What this journey is doing to my life sucks. This whole situation SUCKS! Oh, how my mother despises that word. I heard a great saying: when something sucks, instead you say, "There is no longer enjoyment in this activity." That is great, isn't it? Needless to say, the butterflies in my stomach are now mixed with tears.

As I was telling God in the shower one morning that I wasn't giving up on my healing, the words came to me: "The devil isn't giving up either."

Great! I'm constantly attacked with hurtful thoughts, the prescription always needs changing, multiple sclerosis symptoms are still present, AND apparently the devil's persistence has to be added to the mix of madness. A thought came that God doesn't mess with free will, and I was on my own. No, God doesn't mess with free will, and no, God would never leave me, so yes, my thoughts are being worked on. And in the shower? Crafty little bugger. Is nothing sacred? I love discussing things with God while in the shower.

When I shared this with my friend, Judy immediately started laughing and said, "That's not God—that's the devil. God will never leave you." After backing that thought up with truth from the Bible, that horrid thought never came back. I fought evil with truth on a few attacks and won. Evil hates truth. Fighting with truth is fighting with Jesus. Fighting the devil is not fun, but beating the devil is most excellent. As excellent as that is, obviously I have to watch my thoughts in the shower too.

Was I ever foolish to think my healing would be as simple as taking a dose of medicine. Almost a year later, I find myself working on the prescription and finding it difficult to feel God's amazing love. In my excitement, God's warnings about evil were ignored. I agree with people who say that it is not good to give thought to the devil. True that! We should not give that slime-ball attention, but I personally have learned that it is NOT good to ignore and definitely NOT good to underestimate. People told me not to even mention the devil's name. Name? What name? Anyway, God warns about evil so often and tells us not to be ignorant of the devil's devices. Come on people, only here to kill, steal, and destroy? How much clearer can God make it? If that isn't clear enough, how about God comparing the devil to a lion? God says the devil is as a roaring lion seeking whom to devour. And what? It's difficult to feel God's love? THAT, my friend, has the evil one written all over it. The devil convinced a perfect woman (Eve) not to be satisfied, and being FAR from perfect, Satan is having a heyday with me.

A couple things keep coming to my mind. First is my dislike for believing that my husband is involved with my healing. Why can't I believe my healing is only me and God? The second thing that comes to my mind is: total BULLSHAVING CREAM (thanks, Judy). Isn't the exhaustion from dealing with the strife in my marriage enough? Do I really need to feel more symptoms of MS? I'm still not moved from what the word says on healing, but REALLY? It would be so much easier to give up believing in my healing. This feels like a war.

As I write this, "I'm the victor, and it is so, so sweet," suddenly came to my head. Well isn't that a kick in my butt to take my medicine and keep fighting! The God of the universe is taking time to encourage me! He said I was the victor. How could I ever give up on my healing? No matter how frustrating this situation is, I will not give up. No matter how wonderful heaven sounds, God wants and needs me in this world.

And about that verse with the devil being as a lion—besides giving a heads up, that verse also gives comfort. God doesn't say the devil IS a lion; the devil is AS a lion. HUGE DIFFERENCE! He's just a wannabe. I may get severely detained on this journey, but I'm not giving up.

Recently, God was informed in a rather loud voice that I can't take it. God's encouragement momentarily slipped my mind (all right, may have been slightly longer than a moment). Symptoms appear to be coming as wolves in wolves' clothing. I was being carried if needed, the wheelchair was used way more than it should be, and the doctor was called to begin a treatment of steroids. I really did yell, "I CAN'T TAKE IT!"

This may feel like war, but this is only a battle. And even though it may appear that the devil wins battles, EVIL IS NOT WINNING THIS ONE. I'M THE VICTOR. Because of all the battles going on in my mind, I started seeing a counselor. Sandy is my godsend. I highly recommend counseling (okay, I recommend CHRISTIAN counseling). Rereading how I still wasn't moved from the word concerning my health, my eyes were opened to see that I shouldn't be moved concerning ANYTHING. It's just God giving me another kick in the butt to take my medicine. Or is God helping me only believe? Oh, good grief, WHATEVER!

One day, the word "patience" came to my heart. Really? Patience? I was thinking I'd been pretty patient. Perhaps God knows my issues with perfection and slowness? Perhaps God knows what's going on in my life. OF COURSE God knows. God knows and sees everything. Boy, it is a good thing God is patient and has me covered in the prescription. And it must just tic the devil off that I strive to love with God's love.

Today I find myself with absolutely no desire to take my medicine. Even with signs from God, the distractions keep coming—the blahs are apparently winning. HOLD ON A SEC—God gives me signs to take the medicine? For real, Rhonda? GOD GIVES SIGNS TO TAKE THE MEDICINE! But blah, blah, blah is what I think and feel. DON'T LET THE BLAHS WIN! But what about all the unexplained and strange things that bring strife? DON'T LET THE DEVIL WIN! Why can't I just be excited? GOD GIVES YOU SIGNS! Why can't I only believe? DO NOT LET EVIL WIN! YOU'RE THE VICTOR!

A friend reminded me of my free will. I can choose to let go of the hurtful thoughts that plague my brain or I can let the poison rob me of all that God has planned. Since I want to show God's glory and prove the word, I have to let go of the thoughts that bring strife into my life. The devil losing needs to be a thought that occupies my brain. The devil can't win—that would tic me off. Not letting the devil win should be a huge kick in my butt. The plan to take the medicine and let it flow through my body is back on.

My Prescription

Nope, not yet!

The prescription isn't finished? Seriously?

Today, after reading my daily devotion, I had another defining moment, and this one hit me like a ton of bricks. My trust in God, my relationship, and love for God have to be and come first in my life. It became clear that God is not only helping me write this prescription, He is helping me only believe. With God's love, Jesus' blood, and Holy Ghost power, I'm an overcomer. Oh my goodness, the excitement is back and the blahs have left the building. That may be slightly over-zealous. The excitement is coming back and the blahs are leaving the building—much better. Even though my body feels as if it is slipping away, GOD'S LOVE RULES! I see the weakness as another kick in my butt to take my medicine. I choose to walk in victory. I dare to only believe.

My healing has to be close. I can taste the freedom. Plus, spring is my favorite time of year. I would say that is a perfect time for my healing. Plus my daughter is getting married. I am more than ready to move on in this journey. Before I go, I want to say that I went to a conference for women. God made it clear that the medicine, my prescription, and His word will bring healing to me. God made it clear that loving Him is more than enough. The weekend was exactly what I needed. It got me thinking, why does it seem like there are only Christian conferences for women? Don't men need them also? God says that the man is to be the spiritual leader of the home. Don't men need to be refreshed? It may be easier for most women to get away, but STILL. Dan went to Promise Keepers, a Christian conference for men (is Promise Keepers still around?) a couple of times and came home so on fire for God.

Lying in bed one night, I apologized to God for putting the medicine on the back burner and for not trusting Him. God tells me to do something and I don't do it—pathetic! Once again, excitement has faded into oblivion—so very pathetic.

The prescription is not included in this chapter. I still seem to be working on it. MS is still seen, and there is still strife. However, I do still believe that God will heal me in this present evil world, and in case you're wondering, I still believe that throwing a pair of socks on the floor of a bedroom display at a furniture store would be a great selling idea, as the socks are back to the floor.

Chapter 5

It Was What It Was

Other than working on the prescription, I feel led to add a chapter and call it "It Was What It Was." Not 'It Is,' It WAS! The end has to be near, if not here. I'm beyond being excited. Several events have taken place in my life since those first days. The more major events have been that my dad passed away two years after being diagnosed with lung cancer. Dan had a stent placed in a coronary artery and less than a week later, his dad died in the nursing home. His older brother unexpectedly passed away. Zac bought a house and moved out. Shaina got married to Ben and moved out. We went from having two grown kids and two dogs, to no kids and one part-time dog living with us in the same year. Lucy (Zac's dog) lives here during the week, Zac picks her up for the weekend. Zac says he is breaking Lucy in slowly—it's more that he is breaking ME in slowly. I'm hoping for joint custody. Something I find to be rather sweet is that Shaina and Ben were married on our wedding anniversary, which also happens to be Ben's parents' anniversary. Both sets of parents in first marriages is rare by itself but married the SAME DATE?

Anyway, no matter how much happiness is felt for my kids, no matter how much sickness, death, and free will are part of my life, or no matter how much gratitude I feel to have God in my life, there are still many times I find myself filling with tears. I wanted to make more memories, especially with my dad. I just wasn't done. I WASN'T DONE! I know death is to be expected, but death of a family member is NOT a change I ever gave thought to. Okay, I did think about my kids moving out someday, and they did move out for college, only to move back home again. Did I mention each had a dog? And about my healing, that was expected, of course much different and MUCH sooner.

On my journey, it became obvious that loving God makes life tougher and better at the same time—tougher because of the devil and better because of Jesus. Unfortunately, it was also obvious that, although the devil is down, it is definitely NOT out and it is VERY determined. I often refer to the devil as an "it". I don't feel Satan deserves to be in the same category as male or female. Anyway, the devil's mission was to distract me. Mission accomplished. When I think about all the crappy distractions, it occurs to me that I haven't been loving OR trusting God most in this world. I always thought I was, but nope, I wasn't.

I was talking with a friend about how this world is full of good people doing bad things and bad things happening to good people. We discussed how many people keep loving God despite the bad. I shared the recent defining moment, the hurtful thoughts that cause strife and how exhausted I feel and that giving up, HEAVEN sounds so good. I never gave up on life itself, I just felt like giving up because the fight for my healing is totally exhausting. I'm sick of thoughts from the evil one. I'm even sick of thoughts from the Holy Spirit. I'm sick and tired of it all. I'm not feeling very encouraged today. Many things confuse me. So much happens for which there is absolutely NO explanation. I'm just so tired.

RHONDA, WAKE UP! TRUST THE LORD! OPEN YOUR EYES! STOP LETTING THE DEVIL WIN! WAKE UP! But God, evil is constantly at it! STOP WITH THE BUTS! JUST STOP! PUT ME AND MY GLORY FIRST! JUST TRUST ME! Okay, okay, I'm awake.

My mind can't stop thinking that I wrote that I was even sick of the Holy Spirit putting thoughts in my head. I wrote that? God speaking to me has always been something I cherished. No wonder I can't stop thinking about it. And the prescription was difficult to write because I felt overwhelmed by all the verses I wanted to share. Wait a minute, that's why I said I was even sick of the Holy Spirit putting thoughts in my head—because at that moment, I was sick of feeling overwhelmed. It doesn't make feeling that way right, but it does explain why that was said.

'Blessed' is the way I should feel, not 'overwhelmed'. And why was a King James Version of the Bible requested you might ask? Well, let me tell you, I was led by the Holy Spirit.

Okay, lets just get down to the nitty-gritty shall we? My healing needs to be visibly seen so God's love and God's glory can be visibly seen. Isn't that what this is all about? My healing? NO! God's love and glory? YES (okay, God, you don't have to yell)! God must be so annoyed with me (okay, you do). It is a good thing God is patient. I'm so annoyed with me.

When I began believing for complete healing, there was so much excitement. Both me and Dan were expecting a bow—the bow being an instant healing. An instant healing can and does happen; I have experienced many. However, no instant healing has stuck with the MS. Definitely no bow. Since I believe my healing is a gift, I'm wondering if having it wrapped would be possible. Who am I kidding? I don't need it wrapped. I do need my nails done though. I have an idea. Getting my nails done could be a gift bag for my healing. Gift bags are the way to go. In earlier years, many gifts were wrapped with Band-Aids. Everyone knows if a gift was wrapped by me. The nails being done as a gift bag is a great idea that I am going with.

I was excited to share the complete healing part of my journey with only my husband, but I discovered that that was NOT a good plan. Oh my goodness, believing for my healing is way bigger than either of us ever thought, and clearly me and my hubby are not on the same page. Due to lack of courage, not wanting to rock the boat, or for whatever reason, it became easier to put any thought or struggle that I had on the back burner and just continue working on the medicine. Please don't misunderstand, a person has free will to believe as they choose, and free will is from God. For me though, not being on the same page affects my journey.

It gets me thinking about the story of Job in the Bible. I thought about Job's wife. The story wasn't about Job's wife. We aren't told much about her—the story isn't about her—but what affected Job also affected his wife. They were her children also, her finances also; she had to have been devastated. The only thing we hear about her is that she told Job to curse God and die. Being married, spouses are along for the ride, and what affects one affects the other. As this story shows, husband and wife don't have to believe the same. The story of Job got me thinking that relationships with God are individual. Yes, every road bump hit by me was also hit by my husband, and Dan lives with this disease, but I don't need Dan to believe the same as I do. Our relationship with God is INDIVIDUAL!

After the defining moment and advice to give all strife or any struggle that I may have to God and after the conversation with my friend, my eyes were opened again. I SEE my healing. I SEE God's glory. I WILL PUT GOD FIRST. I WILL TRUST GOD. My eyes are opened. Oh good grief, my eyes are opened again? Time to put knowing into action. Time to be a doer of the word, not only a knower. Not only will I trust God, I DO trust God. I TRUST GOD! I PUT GOD FIRST! The butterflies are so aflutter. Nerve pills, here we come! The more my eyes are open, the more I see! Open your eyes people! What does God want you to see? Though I need a manicure, my heart tells me that my healing will be seen soon—perhaps today or tomorrow—okay, I don't know when, but it will be soon.

As the years have come and gone and as the journey continues, I realize no advice was taken. It may not make sense for most to believe in my healing with symptoms of multiple sclerosis as they are and after all this time, but I will ALWAYS believe in healing, MY healing. God heals TODAY, and God's promises are TRUE. No one will convince me otherwise. Some have tried. Oh yes, some have tried! Anyway, I wake up every morning intending to take the medicine as prescribed, intending to trust God and be a doer, only to become discouraged because of the excuses and distractions. This world IS tough because of the devil, and we need to be tough to fight the devil.

My mind is going a thousand miles a second here. Try to keep up. For this fight I have to be tough. Jesus defeated the devil. Jesus is the Word, which is a sword. I can defeat the devil with the sword. When I take a dose of the medicine God helped me write, the devil is cut. I'm hoping to hit a main artery. This fight can be won. God gave me a sword to help win this fight. I HAVE A SWORD! I know I talk fast. Sorry, I'll try to slow it down. I just saw that the word 'word' is in the word 'sword'—neato!

ANYWAY, a few things came to me this morning. First, I find it difficult to let anything go and get over things. Second, being filled with God's love leaves no room for anything else. And third, reading Psalm 91 on our wedding night needs to be passed on to our kids. I did think about it on Ben and Shaina's big day, but that's as far as it got. Well, they will get it, not sure when, but they'll get it.

Oh, and another thing, cold coffee is a lame excuse not to take my medicine.

I didn't read my prescription once yesterday. Dan and I went to an auction even though yesterday was hot. Heat and MS do not mix for me, but it was still a fun day. It's a shame I didn't take my medicine. Due to the extreme heat, weakness overtook me, and I could have used some joy and strength of the Lord. Those darn excuses. Wait just one minute. It wasn't the excuses. It was ME. I chose not to read a single dose of the prescription. How the devil must have smiled. The demons probably threw a party. It's so clear that the devil's main concern is not my marriage but my healing.

I wish I could talk to my dad. Wait a minute, I can. Excuse me, I need to have a conversation with my dad right now. I love to visualize my earthly father right there with my HEAVENLY father with a smile on his face. I so miss my dad. It will be two years since he died. People always say that it gets easier and the pain will lessen over time. Good grief, I have to wait for THAT too? Both dads are probably laughing at my impatience.

Anyway, as I woke up to another "Not yet" this morning, I realized that I'm fine. I'M FINE! It does bug me when someone says that their trial made them who they are and they would go through it all again. Obviously they found good in bad, or something positive resulted. Well, lucky, lucky them. Personally, not me! I wouldn't wish any part of this trial on anyone. No. Not all people have a positive result or happy ending. Many people become bitter. As I was thinking how someone could say they would do it all again, giving birth came to my mind. It is often a painful experience yet most women forget the pain and have more children. That must be how a person can say they would go through their trial again. They forget the pain and struggles. Because I've got to tell you, being in a trial, the struggles currently are so real in my life, those words would not come out of my mouth. Maybe someday—although I doubt it very much—but not now. NO WAY! I would NEVER go through this again! Anyway, what a different world we would live in if all people brought good out of their trials. I understand why God's word is needed in this present evil world. The devil won't be in heaven. No need for the Bible, we get Jesus himself.

As I was trying to take a picture on Father's Day, my left hand would not stop shaking. My left hand shakes when I use it, but being right-handed, the shaking is generally not a problem. Then again, I discovered that shaking does pose a problem putting on mascara. ANYWAY, finding it impossible to take a picture, we had to ask a person walking by to take the picture. That evening, I went to delete photos taken by me and discovered two perfect photos, no blurry photos. How could this be? I tried many times to get a good picture but my hand shook so badly. While getting ready two days later, it became clear why I had perfect photos. I immediately sent Zac a text and told him we were going to see my healing soon. It may not look like it, but we would see my healing, believe it. I set my phone down totally encouraged that I will be healed on this earth. Yesterday, I tried to take a picture to see if the camera in my phone was just that good. NOT good. The pictures were blurry, and my hand was less shaky than Sunday. It wasn't a fluke. Oh God!

I didn't sleep much last night. I woke up with a hurting heart and the thought that God's love WINS! God's love is ALL I need. I'm the victor. I'm an overcomer! I hear both dads telling me to fight the good fight of faith. People may take that verse differently, but I believe that God is saying that it's a good fight because I win—who loses a good fight? I WIN! My friend Jean asked how the medicine and exercise plan were going, and I texted that, though I'm wising up to distractions, I'm a work in progress. We are talking about my healing and about being obedient to God, and

I'm a work in progress? Thinking how disgusted my response made me feel, the thought came to me that I'm human living in a fallen world. That helped me feel better. But even so, that response is messed up. I know I need to exercise. "Don't use it, lose it" is quite relevant in the MS world, and for me, STRETCHING is HUGE! I know I need to take my medicine from God. Obviously, knowing and doing are completely different. We all know what should be done but struggle with the doing, don't we?

As you read the Bible, imagine cutting the devil with a sword. It so benefits me to imagine cutting the devils wrists. As I was getting ready today, praise music was playing and a pool of blood kept coming to my mind. I listen to uplifting songs about God—songs that encourage me not to give up, lyrics that encourage me to do as Jesus did, songs about God's incredible love. That's why a pool of blood came to me. Praise music also cuts the devil. More evil happened in the world last night. Hold on, Rhonda, a little longer, it's going to get tougher. YOU get tougher, the end of the MS journey is HERE! Keep your eyes on Jesus. Remember He is ALL you need. Hold on, its gonna be a bumpy ride. HOLD ON!

Today I'm feeling a little anxious about the bumpy road. I will hold on tight and do what is needed to keep my eyes on God…whatever that means. Seriously God, what does "Do what is needed" mean? And what does the bumpy road MEAN? I may believe my healing is here not near, but understanding God's timetable is a whole other story. Good grief, I'm so not tough. I never shared with Shaina and Ben to read Psalm 91, and I NEVER took the advice to let go of the strife or any struggle in my life. Oh there's more. Trusting and loving God most was NOT achieved. Is that why the road is bumpy?

God put it in my heart to stop procrastinating. I need to take advice. I'm wasting time. I'm thinking many things are included with what I need to do. A verse in the Bible says that a merry heart is like a medicine but a broken spirit drieth the bones. A hurting heart or strife does not make one merry. It does frighten me a tad how the never-giving-up, at-it-again devil is trying to hurt me. A broken spirit? My spirit does feel like a twig, ready to snap. RHONDA, DON'T LET THAT HAPPEN. YOU'RE STRONG

AND BRAVE. YOU'RE NOT AFRAID. YOU HAVE THE ONE TRUE LORD GOD LIVING INSIDE OF YOU! YOU ARE MERRY—YOU HAVE ME!

While riding my stationary bike this morning, I was reminded of the verse that says, "For as the rain cometh down, and the snow from heaven, and returneth not thither, but watereth the earth, and maketh it bring forth and bud, that it may give seed to the sower, and bread to the eater." And it hit me. That's why I take my prescription. When rain falls on roses, the petals don't break; the rain is good for the flowers. The prescription is good for me. It won't break me. It will help me. I may get confused, but I believe confusion and strife are not from God, and because God lives in me, I will not break. I hear God saying, "Rhonda, Rhonda, my dear Rhonda, this road is long, bumpy, and painful, but you will not break. Give all your struggles to me and always remember that with my love, my blood, and my power, you are an overcomer. Trust me on this!" Yes, God, I hear you— with you I'm tough. I can handle this.

Dan and I have a dear friend who is currently struggling with a serious illness, and we do what we can to encourage and help him trust God. I am reminded daily of how the devil kills, steals, and destroys. God warns A LOT in the Bible about evil in this world. The fact that God gave us armor should be a heads-up that we are in for a fight. It hurts to see our friend struggle with evil taking over his body. A good in the bad for me, though, has been that being alongside Loren on his journey seems to help me on my journey. When I try to encourage him with the thoughts that God put in my heart, I encourage myself at the same time. Another good is that as I share what I write with Loren, a smile appears on his face.

Fight the good fight of faith and God being good came to me quite a bit yesterday. Sickness is so evil—so, so evil. God is so good—so, so good. I am in a God fight. Is my mind ever bubbling. I see myself as having a love-hate relationship; love when God floods my mind, but hate being flooded. The Bible says to abhor that which is evil and cleave to that which is good. I was told to hold on, God wants me to hold on to his thoughts, words from the Bible. I have to hold on to my good, good God. Am curious about something—how do I let everything go? How in the world do I let years of feeling hurt go? Please, God, help me let everything go! And while we're at it, please help me, God, to be finished with the prescription! I'm not begging; see me also as being persistent. Okay, there may be a touch of begging.

I love reading what God had me write. When I write, my fingers just go. I don't even realize what is being typed. Of course, after reading what was written, I often feel like I got my butt chewed out. I've deleted much that was written, because I agree that it's not beneficial to acknowledge or give voice to certain thoughts, but I feel like ignoring makes me ignorant of the devil's devices. Ignoring encourages the devil to act more. There must be a fine line between voicing and ignoring. The thought that the devil is like a chicken, running around with its head cut off just came to me. Hmmm, I'm going to think about that one! I do say the end is here with confidence. I'm not clear when that will be, but it is here though. I feel it!

It looks like begging made no difference, because nothing was let go and the prescription is NOT finished. I have a chicken running around AND my nails need to be done!

Chapter 6

God Loves Me

God put it in my heart that I needed to move on. I'm guessing that God is nixing my plan for this to be a half and half book—half written before healing is seen, the other half after healing is seen. I just felt like God would go with me on this one. It might not be a 50-50 book, but maybe it will be a 60-40 book, 70-30, 80-20…hey, a girl can hope.

I'll begin this chapter by saying that it was quite nice to be informed that the end to living with this dreaded disease is here. Life was hard before, but seriously, the thought that heaven is a place I want to be came oh so often! In a matter of two months, my like-a-brother dear friend passed away. One of my two closest God-friends lost her husband to cancer and the other friend lost her husband to sins of this world. Meanwhile, I was concerned for a much-loved niece who was making bad choices AND Dan's brother and our much-loved sister-in-law separated and are getting divorced. Ouch!

Even though I was told to hold on, I found myself losing my grip daily. I'm feeling exhausted mentally, physically, and emotionally. I am believing in my healing and all that involves, but, oh my gosh, the ROAD BUMPS are proving to be more than I can handle.

WAIT A MINUTE, more than I can handle? Rhonda, don't be such a ninny. God is more important than any trial. People have way deeper bumps all the time—you can handle this. The prescription became my saving grace, and I find that many if not all of my issues and struggles are addressed in the prescription. Boy, I am pumped about my future! BRING IT ON!

Something that should be noted is that when God's medicine is taken, my voice is normal. With the multiple sclerosis, I struggle with talking, but when this prescription is taken, I talk normally. This girl has SO MUCH hope! Thanks, God!

I just had an idea. When something bad occurs, sarcastically say, "Thanks, Eve." When something good occurs, lovingly say, "Thanks, God." Though the multiple issues and the devil's persistence make it extremely challenging, the words are getting in my head and heart.

Hey, I just found something written referred to as "YUK" on the old computer that I'm going to share:

> It seems God is honoring my wish for this to be a half and half book and for me to be done writing, except for working on the medicine—which basically just means changing location of verses and words—which really annoys Dan. I will say that working on the prescription has become more of a saving grace than a curse at this moment. I LOVE working on the medicine. Working on the prescription, I meditate on God's word. I did take a couple field trips—as my friend Rae put it—on my journey with God. Honestly, one field trip in particular felt more like a road-block. Actually, a sinkhole is a much better description. Believing for my healing is the HARDEST and most PAINFUL thing I EVER DID! As hard and painful as it is though, I do know that my healing will be the most rewarding experience I will ever have in this world. I'm not distressed, I'm not forsaken, and I'm definitely NOT destroyed. The Bible tells me I don't need to have those feelings. Well, isn't that just a nice blah, blah, blah. Cause I gotta tell ya, it is hard not to feel that way. With my dad sick, the long cancer diagnoses, my mom sad, my husband often upset because apparently he doesn't understand the situation, it is SO hard not to have those feelings. So I'm gonna ask where does that leave me? I'll tell ya where: frus-

trated and weary. I'm frustrated because I know I should take my medicine—the prescription God helped me write. I feel so good when it is taken. And I feel any delay in seeing healing is about my trust in God. I do feel God's love is all I need. I'm just so tired. I just don't feel like being a winner. I don't want to be a winner? Really? Oh, but I do. I want to be a winner. Besides, my mom and dad, my husband and kids, my friends and family, and my GOD need me to be a winner. I'm a winner when I speak God's word. But I'm so weary. NO YOU'RE NOT! Go take the medicine. I'll take it at noon. I didn't take it at noon, in fact I didn't take it at all. I will start tomorrow. No I won't. Yes I will. No I won't. We shall see. It is tomorrow and I didn't take it, too much going on in my life, I have no desire to take it. I so understand when said the devil loves to attack minds. A mind is a big target. Big and easy target. My mind is attacked daily, and I'M NOT CRAZY!

It has been years since that was written; YUK is right. Multiple sclerosis appears to be taking over my body, and my thoughts about me and my marriage that hurt seem to be taking over my mind. The thing is that the one true Lord God is stronger than the devil, and God lives in me, so that makes ME stronger than the devil.

As of late, a couple of words currently keep flashing in my mind. One is 'now' and the other is the word 'insecure'. This was going to be a 'now' book. I thought I would write about how I was feeling physically and emotionally as I believe and wait for my healing to be seen. I went to the computer every morning intending to do that, but for whatever reason, that was not done. And about the word 'insecure'. Well, after years of persistence and this disease, the word 'insecure' more than describes feelings felt in my marriage. Time to stop feeling insecure and let those destructive feelings go—wasn't I advised of both before? I need to keep believing and trusting God! If only it were that easy; if only it were that simple.

Another word working havoc in my brain is the word 'assume'. I always assumed all would work out. That's quite stupid. 'Stupid' is my word. God's thoughts on the subject: 'that's not smart'. Though being positive is good, assuming often forgets about evil and free will. RHONDA, wake up and smell the roses. STOP tolerating the evil in your life! QUIT being preoccupied by marriage. No marriage or love in marriage is perfect. Only I and MY love are perfect. KEEP YOUR EYES ON ME, AND LET IT GO!

Yesterday, our pastor spoke a message on crossing boundaries. I never wanted to do anything that would 'benefit' the MS. I thought that if anything was done, it'd mean I did not believe in God for my healing. Dan had seen an electric wheelchair he thought was pretty cool. I didn't want to hear about it. An electric wheelchair is something I won't need because I'll be healed. God spoke to me through that message—I was being selfish. This chair didn't have to change what I believed, but it would benefit both our lives (mostly me). Besides the freedom this chair would give, it would allow me the gift of going for walks with Dan and Lucy. That boundary was crossed and on our first walk with the new chair, we saw and talked with friends we hadn't seen for years, and God used those conversations.

One revelation was that you never know when something was said or how your actions may influence someone. I was reminded of the importance of our words. Another revelation was that I did not have it so bad. And it hit me like a ton of bricks that there are worse things that happen in this world. Life could be so much worse and I am blessed. I'm blessed. GOD IS STRONGER THAN THE DEVIL—IT COULD BE WAY WORSE! THE EVIL IN MY LIFE IS TEMPORARY—GOD IS FOREVER! I'M BLESSED—DAN BRINGS ME COFFEE! NO WEAPON FORMED AGAINST ME WILL PROSPER—DAN BRINGS ME COFFEE! GOD IS WITH AND IN ME—I HAVE A GREAT CAREGIVER WHO BRINGS ME COFFEE! Okay, God, I GET IT… my husband brings me coffee. I'm blessed!

Dan and I went away for a couple days. It was so hot. I wanted to be as normal as possible, and Dan was doing what he could for me to feel normal, but it became stressful. Our getaway that had begun with smiles, ended with smiles turned upside down. At one point while at Shipshewanna flea market, I couldn't even operate the joystick on the electric wheelchair. On the drive home I remember thinking, *What is the hold up to my healing?*

God told me, point blank, that Jesus is the cure, and I believe I'm healed. So why is my body slipping away? After making a comment about it being better if I died (because I've got to tell you, as much as I love this life, heaven sounded really good with the day I'd had), Dan's comment was that I couldn't die because a grandbaby was coming. I'm going to be a NANA! And yes, God, while Shaina is pregnant would be a perfect time to be healed.

Sitting by the computer with my 'Nana' cup of coffee, there is much on my mind. I do believe that the end to the multiple sclerosis journey has to be here. God TOLD me that the end is here. I may not understand God's timing, but God, YOU TOLD ME! Why do I wake up with a hurting heart and feel blah so often? Why am I losing strength daily? It is difficult to do my hair and makeup (although I did discover that a little mascara goes a long way, and I love my eyeliner tattoo—thanks, Carrie!) I just feel like screaming; I HATE THE WAY THIS DISEASE MAKES ME FEEL! Never in a million, catrillion, cabillion years would I have thought that it would come to this. Or that believing in my healing would include believing in my marriage.

Oh good grief, I HATE THIS WHOLE SITUATION! People keep reminding me to keep the faith. I'M TRYING, I'M TRYING! Why, oh why, does faith have to be so difficult? I do what I can to cleave to God and resist the devil, don't I? Because the weakness in my body is like nothing I've ever felt before and panic attacks seem to come daily, I'd say maybe not. I just want to live a healthy life with my family and for God. Like I just wanted to shower years ago. GOD, YOU HELPED ME THEN, HELP ME NOW. YOU TOLD ME THAT JESUS CHRIST IS A CURE! GOD, YOU TOLD ME! GET ON WITH IT!

I can't seem to get out of my head that God wanted this to be a 'now' book. A now book? I thought that's what I was doing. Okay, God, you want now? Well, you've got it! I feel terrible NOW! The weakness and the extreme tiredness I feel is close to being unbearable! The strife I feel IS unbearable! My life sucks NOW! Okay, it doesn't suck. I have no pain and I do have a lot to be thankful for. I have a good life! OKAY, OKAY, MY

LIFE DOESN'T SUCK! Although today it feels like IT DOES! Am I done feeling sorry for myself? NO, I'M NOT! I don't want to be a positive role model ANYMORE! I have believed in my healing for so many years, but it's difficult to believe in something when your faith is tried and tried. And the world yells that there is no hope for a cure and there is only medicine to prolong the situation. I don't even have it that bad, and already I have wanted to be in heaven many days. How much longer do I have to wait? How much longer do I have to endure? Seriously, God, HOW MUCH LONGER? God is probably shaking his head and waiting patiently for me to be done feeling sorry for myself. Rhonda, NO MORE pity parties. SMILE and remember that the devil is already defeated!

I was getting ready—or should I say *trying* to get ready—and I'm just going to tell you that there are many days that I do NOT want to be seen in public. People may say that's arrogance, but it's not. I just happen to LOVE makeup and fashion, and I have always felt that it was important to do my best to look my best for Dan and my family. Anyway, it was impressed on my heart that I tolerate this disease and I tolerated this battle and all that includes. Why? I'll tell you why. I'm human with multiple issues living in a fallen world. Presently, I'm finding it helpful to remind God that He told me that Jesus Christ is a cure. I find myself saying 'YOU SAID' a lot. I've questioned God many times when God said to resist and the devil would flee, but the devil still attacked. The devil must not be resisted near enough because no fleeing was done! Discussing this frustration with my counselor, Sandy, helped me see that resisting evil has to be constant. Resisting the devil is not a one-time thing; it has to be moment by moment. Resist the devil MOMENT BY MOMENT—I love that! The devil did what he could to break me and used whatever means possible to steal, kill, and destroy me and the cares of my world. The devil did not give up, but neither did I. I may feel brittle, but I'm not broken. I want to thank God for Jesus, his son, and the Word. I also want to thank God for defeating the devil on the cross, making it possible for me to defeat him. And I need to thank God for my dear friends and all the reminders. God's love is wonderful, and because of our relationship, especially because of our relationship, I didn't break.

So, it brings much joy to say that after much frustration, distractions, issues, struggles, changes done to my words (not God's), cold coffee, paper and ink, and, oh yes, after years and YEARS of tweaking, below are my perfect—to me—love promises from God. The verses are mostly from the King James Version and this medicine may not make sense to you, but it makes perfect sense to me. Really God? Perfect? REALLY! PERFECT! Thanks, God!

My Prescription

JESUS JESUS JESUS This is the day that the Lord has made; rejoice and be glad in it. Enter his gates with thanksgiving and his courts with praise. Be thankful unto him and bless his name. For the Lord is good, his mercy is everlasting, and his truth endureth to all generations. Heal me, O Lord, and I am healed, save me, and I am saved, for thou art my praise. I bless the Lord at all times, his praise is continually in my mouth. Blessed be the Lord, who daily loadeth me with benefits, even the God of my salvation. Selah. Bless the Lord, O my soul, and forget not all his benefits, who forgiveth all my iniquities; who healeth all my diseases. But he was wounded for my transgressions, he was bruised for my iniquities, the chastisement of my peace was upon him, and **with his stripes I am healed.** *Illness is a curse—not a benefit. Christ hath redeemed me from the curse of the law, being made a curse for me. For it is written, cursed is everyone that hangeth on a tree. Let the redeemed of the Lord say so, whom he hath redeemed from the hand of the enemy. O Lord my God, I cried unto thee and thou hast healed me. Forever, O Lord, thy word is settled in heaven. For the word of the Lord is right, and all his works are done in truth. Man says there's no cure for multiple sclerosis, God says there is a cure and his name is Jesus Christ! For there are three that bear record in Heaven: the Father, the Word, and the Holy Ghost. And these three are one. The word was made flesh, and dwelt among us, and we beheld his glory—the glory as of the only begotten of the Father, full of grace and truth. He sent his word and healed me and delivered me from my destructions. For as the rain cometh down and snow from heaven and returneth not thither, but watereth the earth and maketh it bring forth and bud that it may give seed to the sower and bread to the eater, so* *shall thy word be that goeth forth out of my mouth; it shall not return unto me void, but it accomplishes that which I please; it prospers in the thing whereto I sent it.* **With his stripes I am healed.** *Yea, let God be true, but every man a liar. Rhonda, attend to my words, incline your ear unto my sayings. Let them not depart from your eyes; keep them in the midst of your heart. For they are life to those who find them and health to all their flesh. This book of the law shall not depart out of my mouth, but I shalt meditate therein day and night, that I mayst observe to do according to all that is written therein. For then thou shalt make my way prosperous, and then I shalt have good success. But he answered and said it is written that Man shall not live by bread alone but by every word that proceedeth out of the mouth of God. The words that I speak unto you are spirit and life. I don't believe the devils lies, for God is not the author of confusion but of peace. God is not a man that he should lie, neither the son of man that he should repent. Hath he said and shall he not do it? Or hath he spoken and shall he not make it good? Behold, I bring it health and cure. I cure you and reveal unto you the abundance of peace and truth. I restore health unto thee and heal thee of thy wounds, saith the Lord. My covenant will I not break, nor alter the thing that has gone out of my lips. For I am the Lord, I change not.* **With his stripes I am healed.** *I believe the gospel for it is the power of God unto salvation. And be not conformed to this world but be ye transformed by the renewing of your mind that ye may prove what is that good and acceptable and perfect will of God.* **Jesus Christ is Lord to the glory of God, my Father.** *I rejoice in truth—I'm glad. I celebrate in goodness—I'm grateful. I remember to never forget God's benefits—I'm thankful. The all-knowing, all-powerful, unchangeable living word, the all-caring, all-loving active sovereign trinity lives IN me—I'm happy. Heaven and Earth shall pass away, but my words shall not pass away.* **God, I hear your words. I have total confidence and believe your words are true and unfailing. I know you are whom you say and can do what you say. With pure faith and only belief, I speak to every symptom of MS, any malady, and all bad and say in Jesus' name, you're DEAD!** *I had a taste—you ARE good. I choose to act—you ARE faithful!* **I'm not tired or weary—I'm tough and brave. My gut is not scared or troubled—I'm strong and courageous. You said a cure is Jesus Christ. I'm confident and believe that Jesus Christ is the word! With your stripes, I am healed. YOU SAID! You are trustworthy. I'm armed. I'm standing. I say to evil: it is written. There is no room for BAD, only**

GOOD. You took up residence—I'm blessed! I know the truth—you care and love me. I see myself living with perfect wholeness. You told me his name is Jesus Christ. In the name of Jesus Christ of Nazareth, I plead the blood and don't waver. By your stripes, I was healed. YOU TOLD ME! You are dependable! Complete healing is mine! YOU so said it is written God! I believe, therefore I speak. I believe God is big and with me. There is nothing my God cannot do. I'm not scared, I SAID I'm courageous. I believe God is unlimited and in me. Faith in the name of Jesus made me strong. I'm not weak, I SAID I'm strong. **I want to be healed; God is ABLE. I desire to live the abundant life whole; God is WILLING.** Through faith in God I trust and obey. **By his stripes I was healed.** Through faith in God's word I'm certain and sure. With God's wonderful love, Jesus' precious blood, and Holy Ghost's great and mighty power I am healed. **I do ONLY and surrender ALL! God is** the SAME today. Today is this day. I AM completely perfectly totally whole from head to toe in this present evil world. **I'm proof—my dads are incredibly pleased!** I will always rejoice and thank and praise my Lord Jesus Christ. I do so love and bless his name and say to my Lord God alone be the glory. Jesus Jesus Jesus. Set a watch, O Lord, before my mouth; keep the door of my lips. IT IS WRITTEN! I OVERCAME! GOD, YOU PROMISED!

That is just a sample of the prescription—some of the first and last dose. All said and done, each dose is about 12 minutes long, and there are FOUR doses. I told you that taking a pill would be faster. Believing that God wants me to tell you to seek and find for yourself, the location of the verses I used are not included with the medicine.

I sought and found. I found that God's love is wonderful. I found that God is faithful. I also found a benefit with this prescription. With God's medicine, there are no—I repeat NO—side effects! How sweet is that? As multiple sclerosis symptoms are more-than-ever present, I hardly walk anymore, talking is uncomfortable, eating is often something to be dreaded, balance is pretty much non-existent, and I'm always tired to the extreme of having no energy to put on makeup or do my hair. Isn't it time I take advice?

Rhonda, stop being distracted and finish this book!

Chapter 7

What If

As this book is read, remember that we live in an evil world full of pain, but we also live in a good world FULL OF GOD. I am curious about something; what if I were to be successful resisting the devil? What if I knew my only security needed to be in God's love? What if I just cleaved to God and only believed? What if all that were done? There are so many 'what ifs' that I struggle with. Is that why the last chapter is to be called 'What If'—because of my struggles? Or is it because of my curiosity? Didn't curiosity kill the cat? Oh well, whatever!

On my journey, I find it much more pleasant and beneficial to concentrate on God's love and to focus on God, not the problem. As weeds are everywhere, I really do struggle with the word 'control' and feel that people would be happier if they only concentrated on God's wonderful love. I so dislike hearing "God is in control". The thought of God being in control does bring comfort, but we are NOT puppets. And honestly, where does free will fit in with God controlling?! Plain and simple, straight to the point, CRUEL. God is not a CRUEL father. God is a LOVING father—a perfect daddy who desires only good for us. I refuse to see God as a cruel, spiteful dad who uses pain to teach. And really, doesn't believing that God controls everything take any responsibility off us and do just that? I refuse to make God responsible for bad.

I believe that God tries to warn us of the evil lurking and knows how we will handle any given situation, but isn't it up to us whether we hear God and heed the warnings? Isn't up to us how we handle the situation? Maybe it is more than the word itself, so much evil happens in this world because of MAN. We punish those who commit or are responsible for evil, don't we? Nobody likes a controlling person, do they? And concerning sickness: Why do anything and everything to get better? Why not just stay sick and stay in God's will? 'Allow' is another word used. While this word doesn't get me all hot and bothered, the word does bring confusion, and the phrase 'God allows' also makes God an accessory to evil, so I try my hardest to avoid conversations involving either phrase. I feel 'sovereign' is a MUCH better word. God is sovereign. And the word 'loving'. God is loving and 'knowing'. God is...oh, good grief, you get my drift. Let's just say that God has the whole world in His hands. And before I go any further, I want to apologize for the sarcastic alien living in my body who makes an appearance from time to time. Also remember that this book is about my journey, my opinions, and my thoughts and encouragement for others. I've heard that opinions are like noses, everyone has one, and they usually have a couple of holes. Anyway, the way I feel about the word 'control' is my opinion, and I'm sticking with it.

Much to my husband's dismay, the topic of marriage, and our marriage, has become a focal point for years. We live in a fallen world, we just have to be awake to see that it doesn't take a whole lot for evil to work havoc and attack a marriage. All the devil has to do is plant a thought. Go ahead and sin, God already forgave you. Though that thought is true, God's grace gives freedom FROM sin, not freedom TO sin. *The grass is greener, married the wrong person, flirting is enjoyable, want to feel young again, an affair would bring excitement, my spouse doesn't talk that way to me*, are all thoughts that could lead to destruction.

The devil may start the train wreck, but unfortunately, humans have no problem taking it from there. Many get divorced, convinced that life would be more fun with someone else. I feel technology and social media have made sinning easier every day. And doesn't social media bring trust to one's mind? Oh my gosh, there are so many temptations to sin—weeds ARE everywhere! The devil only needs a window open a crack for evil to come in. If you do have a window open, SLAM it shut; lock it if at all possible. And for goodness sake, don't BE an open window.

Anyway, on the way to Saturday breakfast, country music was playing on the radio, and a song came on that spoke of feelings felt in a new relationship or about feelings of a past relationship. I'm not sure, but don't songs like that make a person yearn for passion and possibly encourage thoughts that could lead to unhealthy behavior? Wasn't the devil some sort of music angel? Mentioning the word 'breakfast,' memories come to my mind. Memories are good for your kids and good for your soul; a happy memory is good all the way around. I'm very blessed to have many happy memories growing up. A memory I will always cherish is us girls with my mom, sitting around the table eating breakfast and praying together every Saturday morning before doing chores. The Saturday morning chore thing I tried to pass along to my kids, they didn't bite. I remember my dad getting cinnamon rolls from The Dairy, a local restaurant way back when. As we got older, my sisters and I would meet Mom for lunch, and Dad always had to be with us. We didn't mind, Dad paid. When my sisters and I were married and had children, we would go for breakfast EVERY Saturday. Those memories stick in my mind. ANYWAY, I did find music to be another way evil can work havoc in a marriage. We need more songs that encourage love in a marriage.

I believe on the wedding day couples have full intentions of honoring vows made and plan to stay together, but when there is a glimpse of difficulty, the devil will come in and *WHAM!* Plans change. I feel so sad when Christians divorce, convinced God wants them happy. God does want you happy, but the thing is that God hates divorce, so He can't be happy. Marriage takes work, but isn't God being happy worth it? A spouse not wanting to work on a marriage, heck, DIVORCE has become a norm in this world. It really does bug me when I hear that a divorce took place after 30 years. 30 years? Really? Anyway, not all divorces are the result of a particular sin, and I would never say divorce IS sin, but when a marriage is in jeopardy BECAUSE of sin, I feel mad and sad at the same time. It just seems that many forget about the consequences to their actions—MISTAKE! There are always consequences to sin. Living with guilt is among the many. Guilt often leads to more evil. Some choose to do good because of guilt. More often than not, though, people get blinded by the evil one and think the guilt will be gone if they start over. You may feel like your marriage failed or is dying, but God can raise a dead marriage. Think about and remember the happiness, the LOVE felt on your wedding day. Why become a statistic and go with the world? Go with God!

Speaking of marriage, it has always bothered me that the Bible says women were stoned if caught in adultery. Doesn't it take two to tango? After hearing a message from somewhere, God put in my heart that a woman was created to be a man's helper. So that's why there are so many Christian events for women. A woman needs all the help she can get as how to be a GODLY helper. Another thing that bothers me is when people get married, they stop caring how they look because they HAVE their spouse. All too soon, people appear to forget they need to KEEP their spouse. I'm not referring to changes due to sickness or normal life changes, I'm referring to people that deliberately stop doing what they can to look nice for their spouse because they have one. In this day and age that's NOT wise! Just saying! It also bothers me to hear someone say they feel dumb for not seeing signs their spouse was unfaithful. Could it be they wanted to believe their spouse, love as God loves and endure as God says? Maybe they did ignore roars, but seriously, wouldn't the cheating spouse be the dumb one in that situation?

Upon hearing on the news of yet another horrific story involving sex, it's so obvious these days that people don't care who gets hurt. Oh, I know that sex has been used for evil since the beginning of time and we don't know what goes behind closed doors, but COME ON. THINK, PEOPLE, THINK! A saying that definitely applies is 'THINK BEFORE YOU ACT'. It's BULL hearing all the stories that use sex for evil. God must be so frustrated with this world. And this has to be said: adultery is WRONG for WHATEVER reason. Any type of affair is EVIL. Do not commit adultery is one of the Ten Commandments. It is right up there with killing. That men and women that say they are Christians, yet choose sin over God and have an affair makes me throw up in my mouth a little bit. Think about it; God's law is being broken, that must really frustrate God! And actually, I throw up in my mouth way more than a little bit every time this particular person in my life comes to mind. Oh, come on, my dear friends, be honest, someone came to your mind when you read that, didn't they?! OK, no, that did not need to be said, but I did. Hey, I'm human—just trying to keep it real.

Anyway, I was awoken during the night and reminded that sin opens the door for evil to be active and prayer opens the door for God to be active. Let's pray and let God be active. There is much peace when God is active. Who doesn't love the feeling of peace? And don't let anyone kid you by saying that they are protecting someone by not sharing something negative with that someone. It may be true that they want to protect them from hurt or from worry by not telling them, but aren't they robbing a person the opportunity to pray? It was put in my heart that not sharing is only protecting the devil!

Question: who designs handicap restrooms? What if a person who actually used a wheelchair designed them? The location of the toilet paper happens to be a BIG observation. When the toilet paper is right above the hand bar, it makes it impossible to hold the hand bar. Oh, there's more, why are the soap dispensers so high? I have long arms and STILL can't reach. And WHY are the doors so HEAVY? Even though the wheelchair gives me freedom, my husband STILL has to wait because of not being able to open the door myself and is back to feeling like a waiting wierdo. Another thing, why do people use the handicap restroom when there are regular ones available? Another thing, if a handicap restroom has a push button door that is broken, FIX IT! It was also noticed that in some handicap stalls, the door doesn't close with the wheelchair in the stall. AND ANOTHER THING: 'grandfathered' bathrooms. I understand the reason, but REALLY? For those who may not know what a grandfathered restroom is, my understanding is that whoever remodels an older building is under no obligation to make a bathroom handicap accessible. And especially with older homes, why is the bathroom door the ONLY door too narrow for a wheelchair to go through? What, do people in wheelchairs not use toilets? And why in the world does there seem to be a lip in the doorway to get into places? I need a running start or the wheels need to be straight before entering the establishment. Was it ever discovered that it's easier to STAY HOME?!

What if people took the authority God gave, stopped speaking about the mountains IN their life, and started speaking TO the mountains in their life? What if people didn't grow weary and give up believing for their miracle? What if a person didn't stop fighting for what they were believing for? We don't know what's in someone's heart—they may have reached a point that the fight is exhausting, the devil is exhausting, the waiting is exhausting. Life on this Earth is EXHAUSTING! It doesn't matter how much they love life, they think heaven would be much better. I appreciate that thought because I have been there myself many times. To die is to gain, right? Which brings me to wavering in faith. Being with God in heaven is better than being with the devil on earth. Does thinking that way mean that we are wavering in faith? Faith to be healed? Jesus never told someone to go and pray to be healed, Jesus told them to only believe. Didn't He? I feel a big reason Jesus said to only believe is because God doesn't want us wavering in our faith.

If cures for sicknesses were found and a doctor's office or cancer facility would need to close, I did struggle with the thought of putting people out of work UNTIL a light bulb moment happened. Nursing homes are always in need of help. Should be making last days on earth for an elderly person happy. They have so much love and wisdom to give, so much can be learned from the elderly. My first job was as an aide in a nursing home. Totally, well not totally, I enjoyed that job. It did make for many good stories around the Sunday dinner table. Anyway, I was all excited for the possible closing of a few offices and for any sweet person no longer having a job to find work in a nursing home. I did say 'sweet.' The excitement felt believing in my miracle may have faded a bit through the years, what didn't fade is the feeling that there needs to be more help and more homes for the elderly.

What if prayers were answered the way we wanted? An adorable little boy recently passed away, people were praying and believing this child would be healed, but it didn't happen. Much was done as the Bible teaches, but there was no healing. I'm sure there was confusion and anger along with grief. God totally had the power to heal the child, but the child died. God is not a God of confusion and is there to help with the hurt, but still confusion and pain set in. Why did this beautiful child die? WHY? When I heard that the child's organs were donated, it occurred to me it is possible there were prayers for a donor to become available. It doesn't make one prayer or a person more important or more loved by God than another, it doesn't make the pain less, but it does confirm the importance of praying in the spirit. We don't know all that's involved in every situation, but God does. And for most of us, we don't know what is being said when we pray in the Spirit, but God does. A terminal illness or losing a loved one, no matter what the age, is painful. Advice given TO me during a time of loss is to cling to God. It doesn't take the hurt away, but does help the hurt be more bearable. Advice given FROM me is to remember that 'the secret things belong to God' and to think God believes you can handle this. And yes, clinging to God will help.

What if God opened or reopened a door or window that was shut. Isn't it our decision to go through? Isn't it that free will thing again? For the person who prays for a door to open, I'm sure God would tell you to keep praying. You may have lots of flies in the house when all said and done, but you can always buy a fly swatter. AND PRAYERS—what can be said about prayers that we don't already know? The Bible says pray in the spirit, pray continually, pray without ceasing—do we do any of that? And really, how many times do we get prayed over? When is enough ENOUGH? I started going to a local church for prayer once a month. I made friends and have had multiple WOW moments. God is so there. I always leave feeling so encouraged.

Anyway, a person may feel that everything was tried and the only thing left to do is pray. Don't they have that backwards? Prayer should be first, not a last resort. A person may feel they have no time or they just plain choose not to make time to pray. I feel any excuse not to pray is wrong—talking to God should be a privilege. A PRIVILEGE! God desires a relationship with us. A RELATIONSHIP. It's true that relationships are difficult to achieve and maintain without conversation, but even if a conversation is one-sided, God is listening and pleased with our attempt. So, get praying people. Spill your guts to the Almighty, and get going on the only relationship that counts.

What if we thanked God for removing the mountain before we see it removed? God says faith is being sure of what we hope for, certain of what we do not see. Something currently happening in my life got me thinking that we don't thank God enough. Shouldn't we be thanking God for removing the mountain before we see it removed? I have faith in my healing, but don't see it, and since more symptoms of multiple sclerosis appear, I look silly thanking God for my healing. I shouldn't care how I look. I should be thanking God. And along with being grateful, the Bible says we are to thank God in all circumstances. *Yeah right, I'm gonna thank God for the MS?* It's true that if we look really hard and it may be difficult, having God in your life it is possible to find some sort of good. But as far as the MS? Nope, don't want it and not gonna happen. I believe we should be thanking God IN the circumstance, not FOR the circumstance.

I will say that a good in my life has been having friends that offer to take me to locations my husband would rather not grace with his presence! Dan is great at taking me where I need to go but being a man, the mall is my happy place, not his! I do want to give a shout out to my sister, Rachelle; she always makes herself available if needed. We used to share a bedroom and Barbies, and now she puts my earrings on and cuts my meat. I also want to give a shout out to my mom-in-law. We are and always have been kindred spirits. I am lucky to have TWO moms who love me and whom I love very much.

Here's a novel idea, if people followed instructions. There are many who would rather not be instructed. Maybe it's just me, but don't most men prefer getting frustrated instead of following instructions or asking for help? I feel instructions are there for a reason. Can we get an AMEN to that? The Bible, which is the Word, which is Jesus, is a set of instructions God gave us for our journey through this life. The saying that the Bible is basic instructions before leaving Earth hits the nail on the head. I'm no carpenter, but I do know that hitting the head of a nail is a good thing. Hold on, Jesus was a carpenter, and it's smart to hit the head of a nail. Can you feel my mind racing? God gave instructions to guide us. Jesus was a carpenter, following his instructions hits the nail on the head. Oh, it's racing all right. Here's another good one: a person will often hear that they need to act on their faith. How do you do that? Act on our faith? HOW?????

People are so quick to tell you what you should be doing or how you should be feeling. They have the answer—buy this, do that. Dan and I have become cynical about my healing because of that. I said to Dan that when a person suggests something free to try, that will show they believe in the product and know a purchase may follow. That's why I got so excited about Andrew Wommack Ministries. Besides being a God thing, his teachings are FREE! And it's not just a taste of a message, it's the WHOLE thing. God used Andrew Wommack to open my eyes and see how great the Bible is. My love for God and His love for me were truly blown out of the water. So what if I became obsessed with his teachings and maybe was addicted to how they made me feel! I don't agree with everything he says, but isn't learning more, loving and craving more of Jesus positive? I have a whole new respect for TV evangelists and have many favorites. And I LOVE calling the Andrew Wommack prayer phone line. It saddens me how much negativity surrounds TV evangelists. You don't have to agree with everything—they are human just like us—but Jesus said not to stop someone who teaches or does anything in His name and also told us we should have teachable spirits. Perhaps good resulted from evil in their life, perhaps they hear from God, perhaps they only want to share an opinion and their excitement. Stop finding fault—maybe you too will learn something! It is smart to be careful, but with an open mind and teachable spirit, a person can learn from anyone who uses the Word to guide them. I enjoy and learn from various evangelists and STILL learn. My belief for healing became somewhat buried through the years, but I will be forever grateful to Andrew Wommack for rocking my world and for getting me digging in good soil.

I was thinking about the reactions I received when I mentioned that I believe in my complete healing on this Earth—the looks of pity. People get so uncomfortable. It's unnerving! That should not be, people should be saying, 'Good on you—you go girl!' Being happy and thanking God prior to my healing being seen are more choices to make, aren't they? Good grief, this world is full of choices that need to be made. When I look at my two closest God friends who lost their spouses to fears that have become present in my life, I see how free will and bad choices can and do hurt many people. Both women had undeniable faith their situations would turn around and many prayers were offered, but the situations didn't turn around. Though both women feel sadness, they both made the choice to cling to God.

Wouldn't it be nice to snap our fingers and make the bad in our lives go away? During the night, I couldn't stop thinking of those dealing with a disease and people dealing with addictions. Living with a disease is no picnic, and most addictions have a tendency to take over a life with devastating consequences, BUT an addiction can be beat. It IS hard, but you have a choice. I don't have a choice—wait a minute, maybe I do. I didn't take the prescription that God helped me write. I can't snap my fingers, but I do have a choice. Taking the medicine from God is up to me. I can choose to believe that God's words are true or not; I can trust God or not. I willingly chose not to read it.

I was just hit by more bricks. My poor face; my poor, poor head is getting so sore. My issues are my addictions. Goodness gracious me, I'm addicted to my issues. And trust me, they cover A LOT of ground. So many years were wasted because of my issues. The prescription should have been finished much sooner. I'm quite sure that many would say that mine is no addiction, but I feel great pain in my heart and God said it was.

While having my hair done, Jess made a comment that maybe it wasn't just slowness. Maybe I was choosing to forget why I believe the way I do. Oh my goodness, God, if that is true, I am so sorry. It's even in my prescription that I remember and never forget God's benefits. Boy, does God keep proving himself faithful to me time and time again.

RHONDA, YOU'RE RIGHT, I DO! DON'T LET THE DEVIL STEAL YOUR JOY. I WANT TO BE NUMBER ONE IN YOUR LIFE! MAKE THE CHOICE TO KEEP YOUR EYES STAYED ON ME! DON'T GROW WEARY! CHOOSE TO KEEP TAKING YOUR MEDICINE FROM ME.

Do I even need to say that after many months nothing was let go? I got over NOTHING! I am FILLED with 'buts' and I am NOT referring to a person's backside. A Bible verse says to cast all your cares on God. Blah, blah blah—if only it were that simple. I find myself taking things back and trying to fix things myself—don't we all do that? Being reminded of that verse in my small group, it was abundantly clear of my need for God. And let me just say, if you aren't already and an opportunity arises for you to be in a small group, TAKE IT!

One day, I asked God why I was not only believing. God's response will always stay in my mind, YOU DON'T WANT TO! I don't want to? Oh yes I do, but no, I don't want to be healed without my husband by my side. The past can't be for nothing. God, we have been through so much. You put us together. We are good for each other; we belong together. Not just me, our marriage has been such a testimony. People pray for both of us. Oh, for sure, Dan has made this disease much easier to live with. I'm blessed to have a husband who spoils and chooses to stay with me. Dan's sense of humor and quick wit have provided much laughter throughout the years! I'm very thankful! But God, you know evil has been persistent; the many attacks cause strife and hurt my heart. You know that much bugs both of us and an illness makes everything worse! God, I want to feel like a normal wife. I want a husband, not a caregiver. I do NOT want to live with this disease.

It just occurred to me—I want to stay in my bubble. I want to have my cake and eat it too. God, is it WRONG to like—no—LOVE being spoiled? Is it WRONG to want to stay in my bubble and be healed with my husband by my side? Is it, God? Please, oh, please help me only believe, God. I want to, I really do. And if any unbelief is present, please take that away! Gotta love the persistence with politeness. The devil is not the only one persistent—at least I said 'PLEASE!'

I really don't know how a person can survive this world without God, the one TRUE Lord God OR His word. It disturbs me when I hear that something was God's plan when, clearly, it was a consequence of an action taken by MAN! It is disturbing to hear that a person committed an act of

violence in the name of the god they serve. I feel the verse about God's plan
is used in vain and often used as an excuse to take responsibility off man.
God knows what is needed in each of our lives, and maybe something did
take place that was negative, yet something good came from the negative
and a positive change did result. Personally, I do NOT believe sinning is
God's plan. I believe finding good in the bad to be God's plan! I prefer to
believe God knew I was going to make a smart choice—that was the plan
God had!

I heard a great message in church yesterday. I listened to great teachings
during the night. I should wake up refreshed and ready for battle. I should.
Why don't I? Yesterday I got out of bed totally mad. I was feeling anger at
myself and towards the devil. I was even feeling anger towards God. I was
definitely not refreshed or ready for battle. I am getting weaker and feeling
more tired by the second. This is ridiculous. GOD, YOU TOLD ME!
WHAT AM I WAITING FOR? Really, God, what are YOU waiting for?
WHAT IS THE HOLD UP FOR MY HEALING TO BE SEEN? SERI-
OUSLY THOUGH, GOD. ENOUGH ALREADY! I AM MAD! Then it
came to me—no one is to blame but ME! People may get upset for feeling
God did his part and now it's my turn to do my part, how you feel does not
affect me one way or the other. If there is a slight chance for my healing to
be seen, I'm taking it! What I believe is between me and God!

Oh my gosh, there was more evil last night. There was another disturbing
story on the news. People are SO selfish! I really do throw up in my mouth
way more than a little bit! With all the sin in the world, I understand why
God says to guard our thoughts and watch our words. Most days I wake
up feeling weak and blah! I never did take the slightest chance to see my
healing. No, I did not rid myself of the strife, and no, I don't take every
dose of my God medicine every day. I often get distracted by the attacks
and become preoccupied and don't make wise choices. Taking any chance
to see my healing may not make a difference, but what if it does?

Yes, the Bible is full of questions, but so is this life (thanks, Eve). I have to
remind myself so, so often that the secret things belong to God. This life
is temporary and God has a soft side, and his name is JESUS CHRIST

(thanks, God). It is more than fine for us not to agree on everything—my sisters, even my husband and I don't agree on everything. The way I feel, my thoughts and opinions, will NOT keep me out of heaven, and they give me hope and peace and help me live in this broken world. So, if you have issues with what I believe, it is only something else that doesn't affect me, so GET OVER IT!

I was asked recently what I miss most about a healthy body—that was easy: talking! I miss talking normally. What? I miss talking more than walking? Of course, I also miss putting makeup on and doing my hair as I used to. Oh, how I miss that! I will NEVER believe multiple sclerosis is from God. MY JOY IS BEING STOLEN! Oh, and I miss core muscle strength, sitting in the sun, rearranging furniture, driving—no, I don't miss driving—but I do miss the independence that goes with driving. Okay, there is much to be missed. Oh well, but hey! MY NAILS ARE DONE! In case you didn't understand my gift bag idea, in words you might understand: healing is a gift from God. I do not like to wrap and I like manicures, put the two together, I would like my nails to look nice when I see my healing. Get it? Got it! Good.

When I was diagnosed with multiple sclerosis, I knew very little about the disease and had no symptoms. I never imagined the symptoms would be where they are. I never imagined that I would deal with evil's persistence as I am or that my need for God would be where it is. I really never thought I'd be so in love with God. YES, my relationship with God is above and beyond, but NO, my life is not as I planned. I came to the realization that my dislike for the word 'control' stems from my innate desire for an unbeliever to know God loves them and desires ONLY GOOD for them. So, yeah, I'm sticking with the word 'sovereign'. And it was made clear that God has much to say about our thoughts AND our words. Oh no, here goes my mind again. The devil loves playing games. Mind games are a favorite, and the devil plays for keeps. We get to put on armor. We have a sword with our armor. The Bible helps us win, and God plays for keeps. The game I am playing will eventually be won. Eventually? Whatever, I WIN!

In my discussions with God, it helps to imagine that God is talking to me in a more forceful conversation cause I often need it. Also, many of our conversations do take place in the bathroom ON THE TOILET! Anyway, to think I was extremely frustrated at six months of working on the prescription. It's been more than six YEARS! Who would have thunk it? And working on this book has been like 12 years! Paragraphs, chapters, pages written and lost. Even though I was annoyed with the constant changes to the medicine, I really did love working on the prescription. In fact, more tweaking was done the other morning. Who needs drugs? Working on this medicine gives me such a rush. Being in constant fellowship with God was and IS amazing! That's why the rush: I enjoy the constant fellowship with God, I get it! Don't you just love when a thought pops in your head at the exact time it's needed? 'A mind is a terrible thing to waste' just popped in my head, and so did 'enter at your own risk'. ENTER AT YOUR OWN RISK? I HEAR YA LAUGHING, GOD. YOU THINK THAT'S FUNNY? STOP LAUGHING! I did say I loved it when a thought pops in my head, didn't I? And it's not only God who talks forcefully, so do I. No, God doesn't need it—it's for me!

Oh man, does this disease ever suck! Not one thing is enjoyed. I am dealing with ear infection, argument with Dan, felt attack after attack. I started eardrops for the ear and steroid infusions for the weakness. And what can be said about the argument, nothing to say except 'STUPID'! As I was in the bathroom, feeling tears beginning to form, I could hear God saying 'Those that sow in tears will reap in joy.' My husband had picked up our grandson while Shaina had a meeting, and when Bennett saw me, he would not stop smiling and waving. (Shame on me, I haven't mentioned my precious grandson, every grandparent says theirs is the cutest, but mine IS! Bennett Thor! Oh my gosh, don't ya just love that name?) Anyway, my heart melted and the tears dried up. The love for that child... no words!

After Bennett left, we headed for the hospital, hoping for relief with the steroid treatment. I remembered all the times I testified for God while having this treatment. It began with steroids, it was going to end with steroids. I did have that same thought a couple times before, but this time was different. As the steroids were dripping in my vein, all I could think was I'M NOT CRAZY—GOD IS REAL! THE ATTACKS ARE REAL! GOD KNOWS AND SEES EVERYTHING. WHAT I THINK AND FEEL IS REAL! After talking with a friend, yes, this time was different.

The next morning, I woke up with a smile, but showering later with tears streaming down my cheeks, I thought to myself, *Where did the smile go?* Sitting in the shower, I kept saying rather loudly that I no longer laugh, I cry! The more tears, the more the negative force in my life became obvious. What the heck? It's not suppose to go this way. Negative force? I choose to be on the winning team. I choose to be happy. I should NOT be feeling this way. Evil must be at it again. God keeps telling me to endure, and I'm trying. This whole situation just bums me out. Aren't all things possible with God? YES, THEY ARE.

As I was thinking about God being stronger than evil and all knowing, God cheered me up with His sense of humor and referred to himself as one smart puppy. LOL, I can't stop laughing out loud. God did not stop there. Not only did He cheer me up, He put me in my place. God told me that I was one SICK puppy. God, You stop laughing! It may appear that evil is taking the lead and the devil's persistence is wearing this sick puppy right out, but with God's wonderful love, Jesus' precious blood, Holy Ghost's great and mighty power, that can't happen. I'm an overcomer. Thanks, smart puppy!

Lying in bed this morning, I thought about the three in the Bible who were thrown in the furnace because they refused to bow down and worship a golden image, and how they had faith God would save them, but even if he didn't, they would not bow down to the king's god. I never thought about it before that Shadrach, Meshach, and Abednego were not just warned, they were THROWN in the fire. No matter how scared they were, they didn't cave. They believed the true Lord God, their God, was able to save them.

The circumstances in my life may not look positive, but I will not cave either. Till the day I die I will keep believing that God is able and will heal me on this Earth. If I do die before complete healing is seen, don't feel sorry for me. I have a constant rush. Don't feel sorry for my family either—well, maybe you should. Shaina stopped over the other afternoon, and I was a basket case. She hugged me while I cried and told me that she needed me to keep fighting. I was totally reminded that God is more powerful than evil and that God believes I can handle what's thrown at me. God told me that I know the truth. The ONLY truth I need to concern myself with is that God loves me and God is most important.

We only have one life and one mind, so use both WISELY. God is waiting with open arms! My mind is off to another race. Leap of faith, JUMP in God's arms. Leap, jump. Cool! I do recommend being excited about God. It's also a better way to live. I want to leave a legacy for my grandchildren. Bennett brings joy and happiness to an otherwise dreary life. That sure sounds depressing. I'm not depressed—really I'm not. I have hope. God gives me hope and hope gives me steadfast belief. My life is far from dreary.

Bennett does bring so much joy and is not only the cutest but also the smartest grandchild! One day, Bennett was in the kitchen, there was a toy in the way of my wheelchair. I called Bennett. Mind you, he is only a year and a few months old. He came to me and without even looking at me, moved the toy and went right back to the kitchen. Okay, impressive or not, I shared that because I felt like being a bragging Nana. Oh, and we did get full custody of Lucy, Zac's dog. YEAH!

I do want to share one more special wow moment. There is a magnetic board hanging on the wall by my desk. It is filled with magnets that we have collected through the years that are no longer on our fridge. One is a blue dinosaur. I had been talking to God about how my daughter and husband desired a boy. Shaina wanted to decorate the nursery with dinosaurs if the baby was a boy. The week of the reveal, as I was sitting by my desk, I happened to glance at the floor and saw the blue dinosaur magnet. I picked it up and discovered that the magnetic backing was still on the board on the wall. It wasn't broken, and no other magnet fell. I knew at that moment that the baby was a boy. When blue balloons flew out of the box at the reveal party, I remember thinking, *God not only talks, He listens.* I remember being in the backyard after the reveal just feeling 'WOW!' I find myself staring at the dinosaur still on my desk almost every day.

I will always believe that the will of God is the Word, the Word of God is the Lamb, the Lamb of God is Jesus, and Jesus Christ is my cure. I will always believe in healing and in the sanctity of marriage. I will always and forever remember my conversations with God, the miracles He has done in my life and how, in writing this book, God continued to guide, encourage, strengthen, and protect me. The blahs put up quite a fight—as did my issues and the devil. Weeds are all over my yard, but I'm gonna keep spraying. It was said the prescription was finished many times, but it was not. It was said the book was finished many times, but it was not.

I may never find out if any thoughts were from the devil or the Holy Spirit. It does not matter. Really, God, it doesn't matter? But what about all the strange things and words said that brought confusion and made absolutely no sense? What about the constant need to prove evil wrong or the thought that choosing sin over my healing seems to be a thorn in my side. But God, You said strife hinders prayers.

I SAID IT DOESN'T MATTER—NO MORE BUTS! NO MORE GAMES! Really God? REALLY! THE DEVIL IS PLAYING GAMES, NOT ME! THE EVIL ONE IS TRYING TO CONFUSE YOU AND STEAL YOUR JOY AND STOP YOU FROM BELIEVING IN HEALING. YOU HAVE NO THORN. RHONDA, YOU KNOW THE TRUTH! I keep getting yelled at, don't I? YES, YOU DO! NO, YOU ARE NOT WRESTLING AGAINST FLESH AND BLOOD, YOU ARE WRESTLING AGAINST SPIRITUAL WICKEDNESS. SEE THIS FOR WHAT IT IS. THE DEVIL WILL TAKE ANY CHANCE TO KILL, STEAL, AND DESTROY! YOU HAVE MY POWER INSIDE YOU! YOU TAKE ANY CHANCE. DO NOT LET THE EVIL WIN!

I can't stress enough how important our thoughts and words are. Or stress that we should never stop praying. To pray continually goes without saying. To pray without ceasing, I feel means DON'T GIVE UP! So, no, NEVER stop praying. NEVER stop believing. NEVER stop fighting! The devil won't quit, so why should you? NEVER GIVE UP ON GOD! God won't quit either.

If anything in this book made you feel like I was telling you what to do, that was not my intention. It is also not my intention for you to feel judged or feel bad. What a person did and where a person is at in their belief is between them and God! My intention is to encourage and perhaps inspire you in some way and to share my excitement about what I learned that helped me on my journey in this life. What we believe and how we think DOES impact our lives. Don't let theology or growing up with 'religion', or any other past or present experience define you or the way you think. Read the Bible for yourself, and let God's love define you. Let GOD define you. Maybe I am telling you what to do.

There are many who have happy memories, happy lives, and have found peace in a trial and use their trial to bring God glory. And there are so many worse things that happen in this world. We all have had loved ones get sick and die, accidents happen, divorce happens, much sadness takes place in this world even when prayer and faith were in abundance. I know all this. I know there are many way more excited about God and I'm not the only person to hear God's voice. I'm sure you have your own 'what if's and questions. I'm sure you have your own opinions and words of wisdom. If you are going through something painful, I'm sorry! Whatever your journey, make the choice and choose God. Read the word in any version and diligently seek God. Use the Bible to guide you and talk to God about everything and back up any thought with the Bible. You can't lose with the one TRUE Lord God on your team.

This past weekend I was reminded that sad things happen! We question God—the questions are endless. I wonder what are You thinking?!?! I keep hearing God whisper, *This life is just temporary...this life is just temporary... this life is just temporary.* This life is temporary, and wherever your life takes you, with God you can handle it!

My book includes thoughts, opinions, and many memories. I am just a regular person who has made her share of mistakes. My mind bounces all over the place and goes from one thought to another in an instant. I repeat and say 'anyway' A LOT. Sometimes I say something completely random (boy, that bugs my husband). Sometimes I make no sense (boy, that bugs my husband too). I shared many conversations with God. I shared many thoughts on marriage and God let me go. I was honest—nothing was sugar-coated, maybe deleted, but not sugar-coated! I wrote how important the Word is and how persistent and determined the devil is. "Okay, God… Really?" is a question multiple times DAILY.

Hopefully I got your mind going and gave you something to think about and at some point put a smile on your face. I said that books upon books were written; there are many books with great advice and helpful ideas written, many memoirs with much good but with no God. Well, not mine—God's all over mine!

No, my life did not go as planned, but yes, I will forever choose God and choose to be happy. Feeling that God is pleased with me makes me happy. Honestly, God gets me through each and every day. This life gets confusing, and we all have questions. But we can have peace knowing the secret things belong to God and believing the Word, Jesus Christ, that the one true Lord God is not the liar. I don't know what the future will bring. I know complete healing is not just about the multiple sclerosis in my body and that I need to keep enduring. Me, my family, and this marriage have been through way too much, and I have come too far to give up now. I will say that evil persistence was and is extremely rough on my marriage; the devil's sheer determination that I felt would be rough for any marriage. I never saw any of this coming. I keep telling myself that this too shall pass. I'm going to stand firm in my belief for healing, stock up on insect repellent, and bask in God's love. I will not cease in my praying for complete healing! I'm way, WAY past letting evil win! God's glory WILL be seen!

I want to speak to those directly affected with multiple sclerosis, don't look at me and worry that you'll end up in a wheelchair—don't let that frighten you! 'You have nothing to fear but fear itself' is another saying that starts the engines. Really though, tightness felt in my legs has been a huge problem with my ability to walk. I advise stretching exercises. When your mind tells you not to do something, do it anyway. That's been my case. I also advise smiling! Being greeted with a smile totally impacts the way you feel. It should be a smile a day keeps the doctor away.

God telling me this book was written for me is all fine and dandy, and there are lots of reasons it could have been written, but I'm holding out for people needing good. There is so much more that I could say, but I will stop with this: THINK GOOD, POSITIVE THOUGHTS AND GUARD THEM. WATCH WHAT YOU SAY. MAKE SMART CHOICES. CHOOSE TO BE HAPPY WHERE YOU ARE! BE AWARE OF EVIL'S DETERMINATION, AND KEEP ENDURING. PRAY ABOUT EVERYTHING AND ALWAYS REMEMBER THAT YOU HAVE NOTHING TO LOSE AND EVERYTHING TO GAIN! DON'T EVER STOP BELIEVING.

This book may not end with seeing a healing, but I will not stop praying, believing, trusting, and loving as God loves. I'm going to walk by faith fully armed with a smile on my face and bug and weed spray in my hand. I'm going to take the prescription God wrote with me, work on taking advice, and see what happens.

God wants you to know that you are always a winner in His book. Read it and allow God the opportunity to be life and health on your journey. Allow yourself the opportunity to fall more in love with God. It's time for me to pull weeds and be courageous. It's time to trust and obey God, moment by moment. I could go on and on. I won't though, BUT I'm also gonna stop with this thought from God: recognize and give thanks for the wow moments. With the one true Lord God constantly speaking, I'm not just running, I'm sprinting. Put on your running shoes. Let's cross the finish line together.

It's been nice chatting with you. And for whatever reason if it may have been needed, I do hope you were encouraged! Sorry if I talked your ear off; it will grow back. Hopefully no one was lost by the wayside by how my mind works. Maybe we will meet in person someday. Try not to look too close, and I will try not to repeat, ramble, or talk fast—not promising anything, but I will try.

My journey with the prescription did come to an end. My journey with this book is coming to end. My journey with multiple sclerosis will come to an end. My journey with God...that, my friend, is just beginning.

My journey to complete healing...to be continued!

As I was looking at pictures to include in this book, I was brought to such a happy place in my heart. I was reminded how blessed I feel that I was able to be a regular mom while Zac and Shaina were growing up. I thought of all the good times and found so many wonderful photos I wanted to share. Here are just a few to help you put a face to what was read.

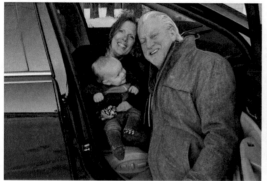

▲ "I love how Bennett is looking at his Papa. We had just gotten home from Bennett's 1st birthday party, and I realized that I had no picture with him on his 1st birthday, so I had Dan get up from the couch, get me back in the car and drive to Shaina's house. I waited in the car, and Shaina brought Bennett out so I could get my picture."

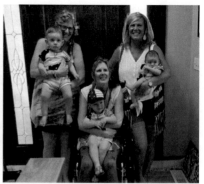

▲ "Me and my sisters became first-time nanas within a year and a half of each other. ALL BOYS!"

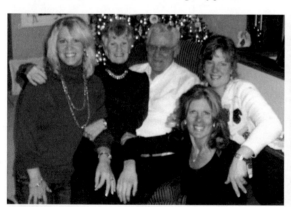

▲ "The original five DeHaan family—my sister Rachelle, my mom and dad, my sister Robin, and myself!"

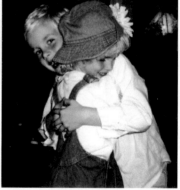

▲ "One of my favorite pictures of Zac and Shaina. I hear stories about how the sibling love may have been misplaced for a few years, but I will always have my pictures!"

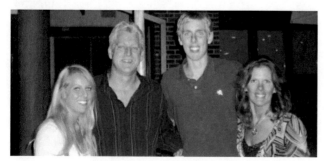

◀ "Celebrating a birthday. See how tall Zac got? Good thing he doesn't drop me!"

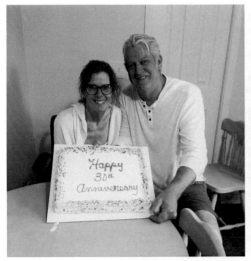

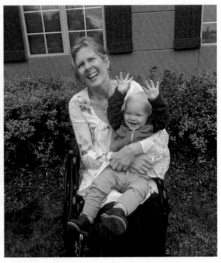

▲ "I thought we were going to hang out with Shaina and Ben because we share anniversaries. Instead, the kids threw a surprise party for us! They indeed pulled it off! I was not dressed for a party—little makeup, glasses not contacts, hair a mess, and no bra. SURPRISE!"

▲ "Bennett is not replacing Zac and Shaina, but with them being so big, Bennett is much cuter doing so big!"

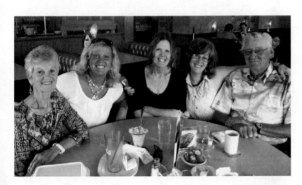

◄ "Us girls having lunch together. Yep, Dad had to be there."

"Us girls still meet for lunch whenever we can. Even without Dad" ►

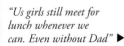

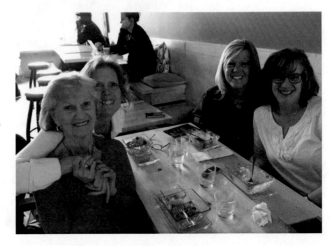

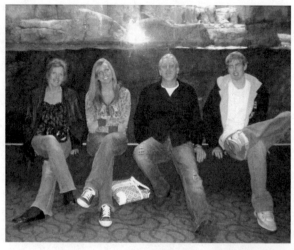

◀ *"Relaxing on vacation."*

"Our Christmas photo—Lucy's eyes look possessed but at least my feet were warm!" ▼

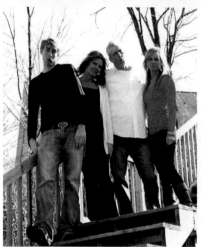

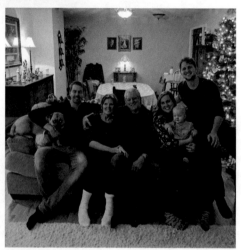

▲ *"I may not be normal, but neither is my family!"*

"The last picture on Christmas Eve with my dad. He died a few months later." ▶

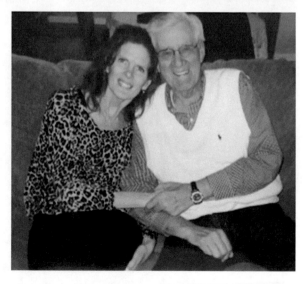

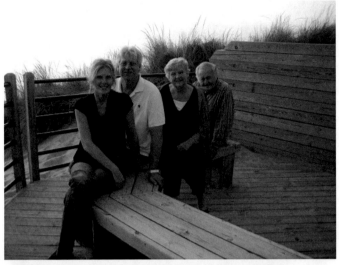

◀ *"This is a special photo with special people at a special place. Me and Dan with his mom and dad on the anniversary of the day Dan's brother, Jeff, passed away."*

"Bennett looking at me so intently. He was probably shocked that his nana had no makeup on and her hair was not done" ▼

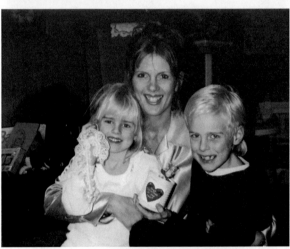

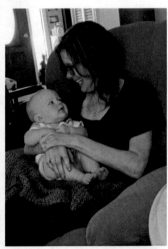

▲ *"A picture taken around the time I was diagnosed with MS."*

"Our wedding. Looking into each other's eyes with so much love, not giving thought to the vows we were about to make to each other or the journey that we were about to embark on. I had optic neuritis a few months later." ▶

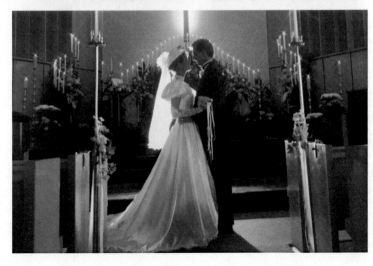

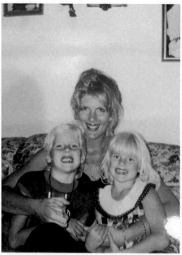

▲ "I adore this picture! Can't ya just feel the love?

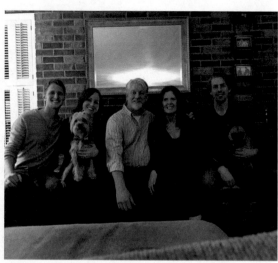

▲ "Lucus (Shaina's dog) and Lucy (Zac's dog) became part of this family for sure! Along with Ben, my favorite son in law who always has my back!"

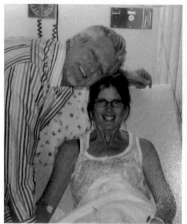

▲ "It must have been a God week—I allowed a picture to be taken at the hospital!"

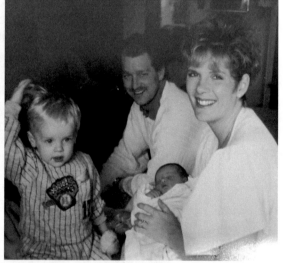

"I had my Shaina!" ▲

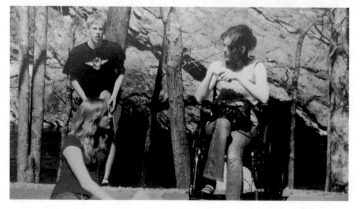

◄ "The holes in my jeans and being in a wheelchair didn't stop us from having a great vacation!"

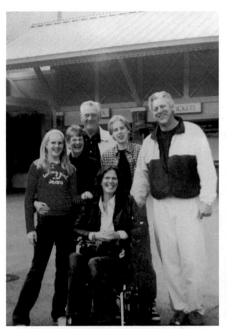

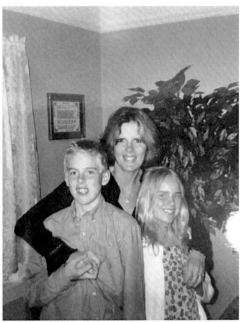

▲ *"When the kids were in grade school, my parents began going to Tennessee for a month every year, and we would go for a week every year to see them. The wheelchair was positively my gift from God. Many awesome memories!*

▲ *"My heart smiles at this picture!"*

"A special picture I've kept framed and in my family room for over 25 years. Zac and Shaina feeding the ducks at SeaWorld before our lives changed!" ▼

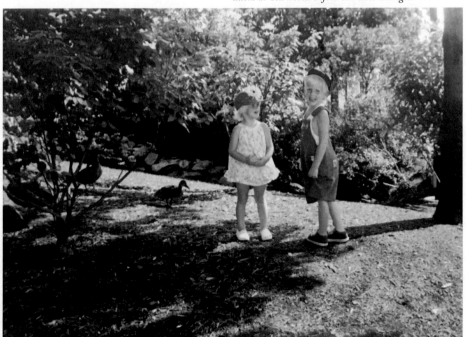

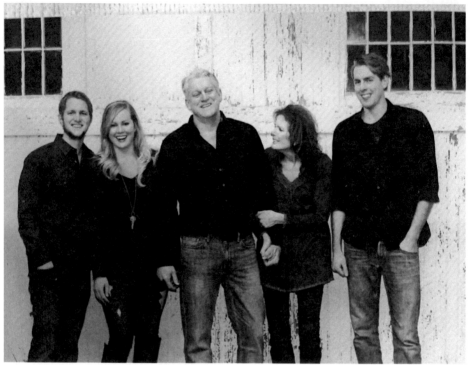

▲ "Having family pictures taken at a friends farm."

"Our yearly vacation to the Smokey Mountains." ▼

"So grateful I was able to be a regular wife and mom!" ▼

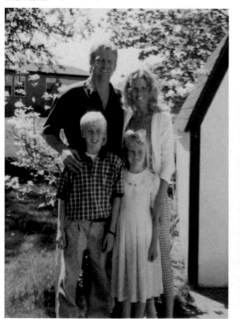

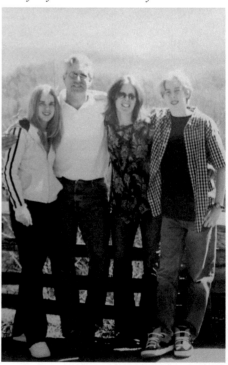

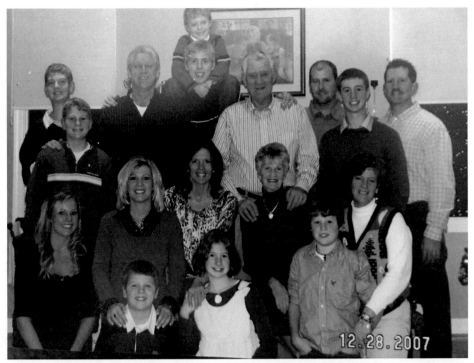

▲ "I had to include an annual Christmas photo of the original 17 DeHaan family.

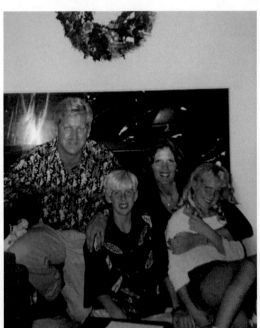

▲ "Another photo that makes my heart smile, I don't even think about what tomorrow might bring."

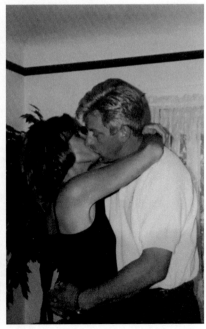

▲ "The memories are endless! Our life did not go as planned, but our children, our love, our GOD are worth it! I will not give up—I will keep fighting. Where's my sword?"

Acknowledgments

First and foremost, my biggest acknowledgment is to our Almighty God, my co-author. Thank you for the daily encouragement to keep writing and keep believing in my healing. Thank you also for all the wow moments throughout the years. You never left my side and stuck to me like glue! I will always love and praise You, God, no matter what!

I want to thank my husband for doing everything possible to make my life easier while I wrote this book. It was not a simple task dealing with evil persistence on a daily basis, not fully understanding the situation, and not seeing eye to eye, but you still brought me coffee every day and put up with the issues that were thrown at us! Thank you for believing with me that all things are possible with God. I'm grateful we chose each other to do life together. Thank you for taking such good care of me and for letting me stay in my bubble.

I want to thank Zac and Shaina for giving me great stories and precious memories. I'm honored and privileged to be your mom. Thanks for putting up with any annoyance you endured while growing up and for handling things so well. Thank you for being you!

I want to thank all the friends who encouraged and prayed for me, and my hubby through the years. To my friends who stayed with me, you know who you are—thank you so much! And a special thank you to my dear friend Pat, another constant in my life; you would not let me give up writing this book, and you did your best to keep the sarcastic alien at bay and not offend anyone. I'm sorry if I stepped on any toes.

Oh, and I can't forget to thank Katie, my project manager and editor. With me feeling like I had to run everything past God, my mind as it is, and with the multiple sclerosis symptoms on top of that, dealing with me has been more than a little challenging to say the least. Thank you for being so patient and understanding! I so need to thank you, Atlantic Publishing, for giving me—an unknown, regular person who wrote a book—a chance.

I also want to thank God for the armor supplied, and a personal thanks goes to all who continue to pray for me and Dan on a daily basis. Thank you, thank you, THANK YOU!

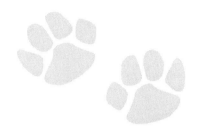
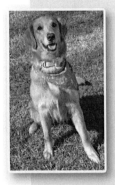
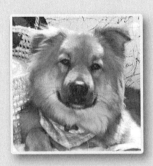
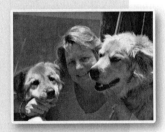

Over the years, we have adopted a number of dogs from rescues and shelters. First there was Bear and after he passed, Ginger and Scout. Now, we have Kira, another rescue. They have brought immense joy and love not just into our lives, but into the lives of all who met them.

We want you to know a portion of the profits of this book will be donated in Bear, Ginger and Scout's memory to local animal shelters, parks, conservation organizations, and other individuals and nonprofit organizations in need of assistance.

– Douglas & Sherri Brown,
President & Vice-President of Atlantic Publishing